PROBLEM-BASED OBSTETRIC ULTRASOUND

PROBLEM-BASED OBSTETRIC ULTRASOUND

Basky Thilaganathan MD MRCOG
Consultant and Director
Fetal Medicine Unit
St George's Hospital Medical School
London
UK

Shanthi Sairam MD MRCOG
Senior Clinical Fellow
Fetal Medicine Unit
St George's Hospital Medical School
London
UK

Aris T Papageorghiou MRCOG
Consultant Maternal-Fetal Medicine
Fetal Medicine Unit
St George's Hospital Medical School
London
UK

Amar Bhide MD MRCOG
Consultant Maternal-Fetal Medicine
Fetal Medicine Unit
St George's Hospital Medical School
London
UK

informa
healthcare

Informa Healthcare USA, Inc.
52 Vanderbilt Avenue
New York, NY 10017

Visit the Informa Web site at
www.informa.com

and the Informa Healthcare Web site at
www.informahealthcare.com

CONTENTS

FOREWORD

This short textbook on problem-based obstetric ultrasound is an important and needed text for those who scan for fetal anomalies. The book takes a pragmatic approach by first defining an anomaly followed by a decision tree that indicates what other features need to be investigated to reach the definitive diagnosis. In a short text it is difficult to cover the entire pathology seen on scanning, but it covers more than adequately most of the common problems.

In addition to the decision algorithms, the text is well illustrated by the appropriate scan pictures which would be of immense value.

I am delighted that such a book is produced at last by a team of four experts in the field of fetal medicine.

Sabaratnam Arulkumaran
Professor and Head, Obstetrics and Gynaecology
St George's University of London
London

1

VENTRICULOMEGALY

The lateral cerebral ventricles are best measured in that part of the posterior horn at the level of the choroids plexus (atrium). The following terminology is followed most often:

- normal: measurement < 10 mm
- mild/borderline ventriculomegaly: 10–12 mm
- moderate ventriculomegaly: 12–15 mm
- severe ventriculomegaly: > 15 mm.

In the majority of cases, the outcome is good for isolated mild/borderline or unilateral ventriculomegaly, suggesting that it is a normal variant. When the ventriculomegaly is bilateral or the measurement is above the 97.5th centile (> 12 mm), the neonatal outcome is associated with the cause of the ventriculomegaly rather than the amount of fluid in the ventricle.

Aneuploidy

Advanced maternal age, high risk screen test results, or the presence of other ultrasound markers of chromosomal abnormality should raise the possibility of fetal aneuploidy. Typically, aneuploidy, if present, is associated with mild rather than moderate or severe ventriculomegaly.

Congenital viral infection

Although rare, the presence of ultrasound features confers a terrible prognosis for congenital fetal viral infection. Typical ultrasound features include severe fetal growth restriction, microcephaly, focal brain hyperechogenicities, and cardiac abnormalities.

Brain haemorrhage

Clots are rarely seen on fetal brain ultrasound, but if seen are characteristic of intracerebral bleed as a cause. In the absence of such a finding, parental blood should be taken to exclude the possibility of fetal alloimmune thrombocytopenia.

Structural brain abnormality

The finding of other structural brain abnormality generally confers a poor neonatal prognosis. The exceptions to this rule are arachnoid cyst (see 'Intracranial cysts') and isolated agenesis of the corpus callosum with normal gyral development.

Bibliography

1. Gaglioti P, Danelon D, Bontempo S et al. Fetal cerebral ventriculomegaly: outcome in 176 cases. Ultrasound Obstet Gynecol 2005; 25(4): 372–7.
2. Laskin MD, Kingdom J, Toi A, Chitayat D, Ohlsson A. Perinatal and neurodevelopmental outcome with isolated fetal ventriculomegaly: a systematic review. J Matern Fetal Neonatal Med 2005; 18(5): 289–98.

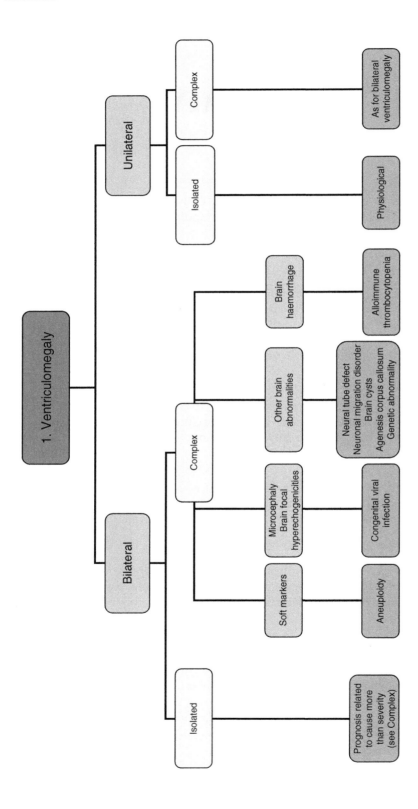

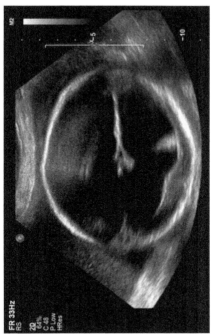

Fig. 1.2 *Severe ventriculomegaly*

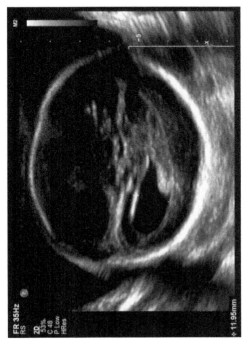

Fig. 1.1 *Moderate ventriculomegaly*

2

INTRACRANIAL CYSTS

The origins of intracranial cysts are best identified by their position and associations within the brain as outlined in the diagnostic algorithm.

Choroid plexus cysts

These are collections of the cerebrospinal fluid (CSF) due to blockage of the glands in the choroids plexus. They are seen in 1–3% at the time of the anomaly scan, and occur most commonly in the lateral ventricles. In the absence of associated ultrasound features of fetal aneuploidy, the outlook for the pregnancy is good, with natural resolution in pregnancy being the inevitable outcome.

Arachnoid cysts

These are rare cysts arising from the arachnoid membrane. They are most often isolated, regular, and non-midline, and the size can be very variable. Midline shift of the brain may be seen due to the pressure effect. The outlook is usually good, unless the size is extraordinarily large.

Inter-hemispheric cysts (pseudocysts)

The ultrasound appearance is of a cystic structure in the midline, and they are often mistaken for arachnoid cysts. These pseudocysts result as a consequence of a deficiency in the roof of the third ventricle and agenesis of the corpus callosum. The outlook is guarded because of the structural brain abnormalities associated with this finding.

Posterior fossa cysts

These are variably (and confusingly) termed Dandy–Walker cysts, variant, or malformation. In practical terms it is better to describe the ultrasonographic findings, i.e. posterior fossa cyst with/without agenesis of the cerebellar vermis. The outlook is generally guarded if there is total agenesis of the vermis or the cerebellum is hypoplastic. The prognosis may be good in some cases of apparent partial agenesis of the vermis, due to rotation rather than agenesis of the vermis.

Vascular malformations

Aneurysm of the vein of Galen and dural sinus malformations are rare diagnoses easily made by the use of colour Doppler interrogation of apparent cystic masses in the brain. The prognosis for a vein of Galen malformation is good in the absence of fetal hydrops. In contrast, poor neurodevelopmental outcomes have been reported for dural sinus malformations.

Bibliography

1. Blaicher W, Prayer D, Bernaschek G. Magnetic resonance imaging and ultrasound in the assessment of the fetal central nervous system. J Perinat Med 2003; 31(6): 459–68.
2. Pilu G, Visentin A, Valeri B. The Dandy-Walker complex and fetal sonography. Ultrasound Obstet Gynecol 2000; 16(2): 115–17.

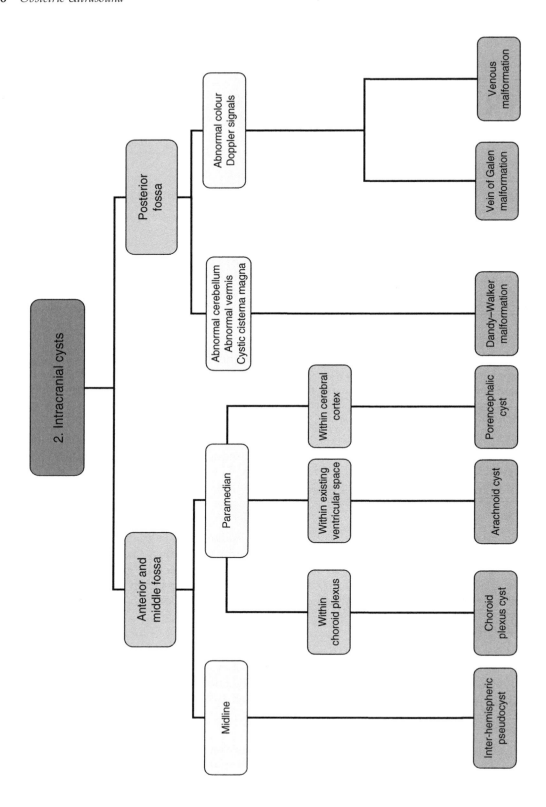

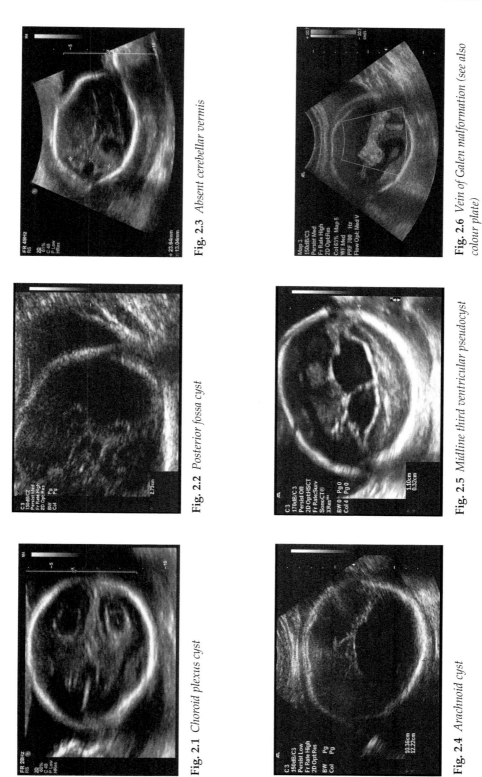

Fig. 2.3 *Absent cerebellar vermis*

Fig. 2.6 *Vein of Galen malformation (see also colour plate)*

Fig. 2.2 *Posterior fossa cyst*

Fig. 2.5 *Midline third ventricular pseudocyst*

Fig. 2.1 *Choroid plexus cyst*

Fig. 2.4 *Arachnoid cyst*

3

ABNORMAL SKULL SHAPE

Abnormalities in skull shape are relatively rare, but quite striking when seen. An ability to recognize the described shapes is invaluable in the diagnosis of the aetiology and associated abnormalities.

Lemon shaped skull

This is a characteristic feature of spina bifida, often associated with a 'banana' shaped cerebellum due to herniation of the cerebellar vermis through the foramen magnum. The lemon shape is most often seen in the middle third of pregnancy, and often resolves in the third trimester. 'Lemon-like' skull without spina bifida has no clinical significance, and therefore a careful search of the spine is indicated before disregarding this finding.

Strawberry shaped skull

This finding should raise the suspicion of trisomy 18 (Edward syndrome). A careful examination should be conducted to exclude other markers of chromosomal abnormality (choroid plexus cysts, ventriculomegaly, clenched fists, congenital heart disease, congenital diaphragmatic hernia, exomphalos, single umbilical artery, and talipes).

Clover-leaf shaped skull

This is typically associated with skeletal dysplasias. Hence, associated findings are shortening of the long bones and narrowing of the chest (thoracic dysplasia) such that the heart appears to fill more of the chest (apparent cardiomegaly).

Encephalocele

The prognosis is generally poor unless the defect contains only meninges without brain matter. When an occipital encephalocele is diagnosed, an effort should be made to exclude Meckel–Gruber syndrome (occipital encephalocele, polycystic kidneys, polydactyly), which has an autosomal recessive pattern of inheritance.

Achondrogenesis

This is a skeletal dysplasia where the skull is very poorly mineralized, and easily deformed by the pressure of the ultrasound probe.

Bibliography

1. Glass RB, Fernbach SK, Norton KI, Choi PS, Naidich TP. The infant skull: a vault of information. Radiographics 2004; 24(2): 507–22.
2. Lachman RS, Rappaport V. Fetal imaging in the skeletal dysplasias. Clin Perinatol 1990; 17(3): 703–22.

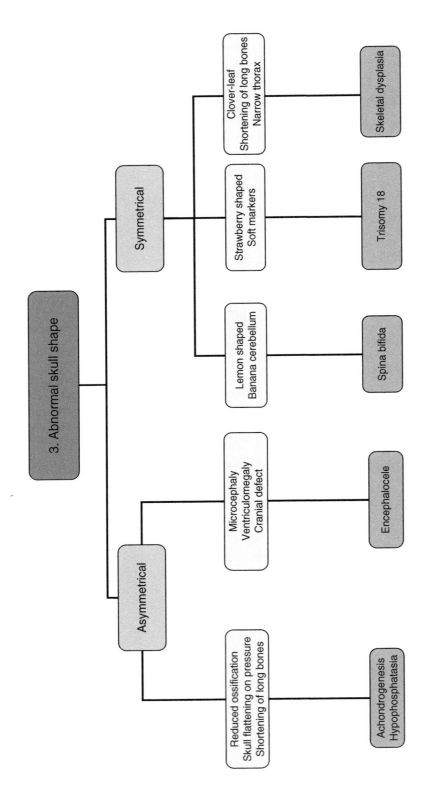

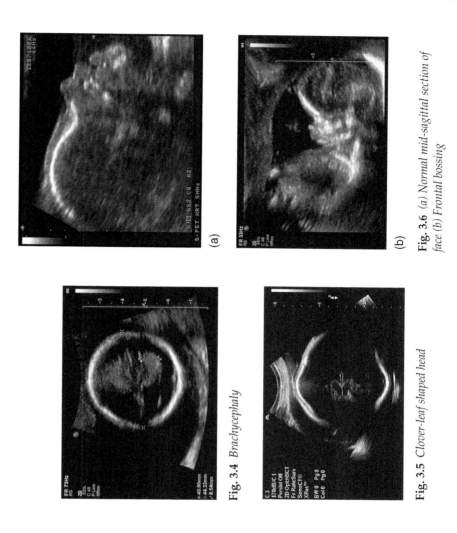

Fig. 3.6 *(a) Normal mid-sagittal section of face (b) Frontal bossing*

Fig. 3.4 *Brachycephaly*

Fig. 3.5 *Clover-leaf shaped head*

Fig. 3.1 *Lemon shaped head*

Fig. 3.2 *Banana cerebellum*

Fig. 3.3 *Strawberry shaped head*

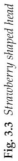

4

FACIAL CLEFTS

Ultrasound recognition of facial clefts involves obtaining a coronal surface view of the face showing the lips and nostrils. The defect in the alveolar ridge is demonstrable on a transverse view (often mistaken for the primary/hard palate). A profile view may demonstrate a pre-maxillary protrusion in cases of bilateral cleft lip/alveolus. The primary palate is not normally visualized on ultrasound. The defect of the alveolar ridge can be demonstrated by, and in most cases is associated with, a defect of the primary palate. Prenatal diagnosis of cleft palate in the absence of a cleft lip/alveolus is extremely difficult. Recently, the use of 'reverse face view' on three-dimensional ultrasound has been described to improve prenatal identification of defects of the palate.

Facial clefts are typically an isolated finding, but may have a group of conditions associated with them. Median and bilateral facial clefts are associated with a higher risk of underlying chromosomal (trisomy 13) or genetic abnormality. The commonest genetic syndromes typically involve either midline defects of the brain (holoprosencephaly) or defects of the somatic structures. Clefts (usually of the palate) are commonly associated with some craniosynostoses.

Bibliography

1. Campbell S, Lees C, Moscoso G, Hall P. Ultrasound antenatal diagnosis of cleft palate by a new technique: the 3D 'reverse face' view. Ultrasound Obstet Gynecol 2005; 25(1): 12–18.
2. Wayne C, Cook K, Sairam S, Hollis B, Thilaganathan B. Sensitivity and accuracy of routine antenatal ultrasound screening for isolated facial clefts. Br J Radiol 2002; 75(895): 584–9.

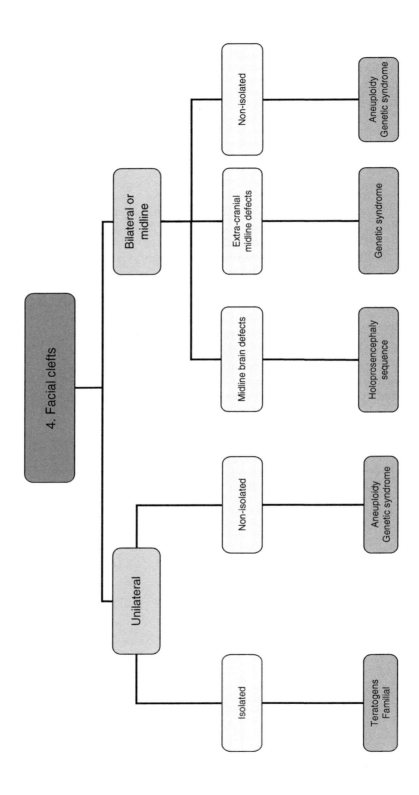

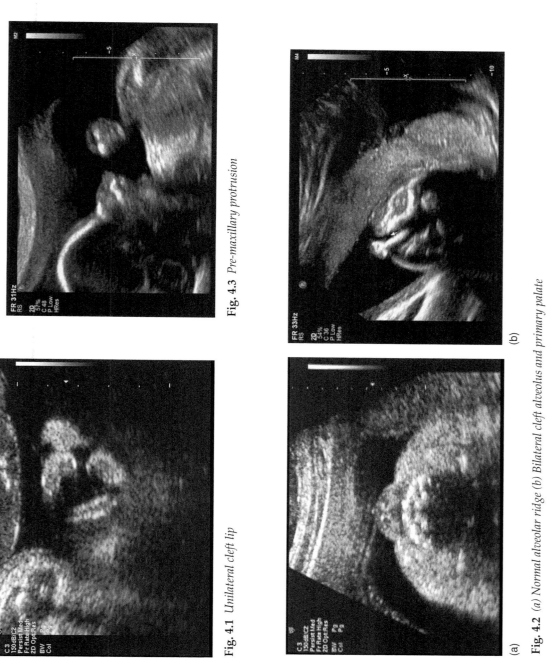

Fig. 4.1 *Unilateral cleft lip*

Fig. 4.3 *Pre-maxillary protrusion*

(a)

(b)

Fig. 4.2 *(a) Normal alveolar ridge (b) Bilateral cleft alveolus and primary palate*

5
ABSENT NASAL BONES

The association of nasal bone hypoplasia and trisomy 21 is now well established. There are ultrasound studies in low-risk and high-risk populations, and also histopathological studies in fetuses with Down syndrome, which have consistently confirmed this association. Some 50–60% of fetuses with Down syndrome will have absent nasal bones at 11–14 weeks on ultrasound scanning. However, nasal bones may be absent in a small proportion of chromosomally normal fetuses as well. The background prevalence of absent nasal bones in normal fetuses is dependent on the parent's ethnicity and facial structure.

Advanced maternal age, increased nuchal translucency, abnormal serum biochemistry, and abnormalities or soft markers seen on ultrasound are the factors to be considered in determining the a-priori risk for trisomy 21. Absence of the nasal bones would significantly increase the chance of underlying trisomy 21, and an invasive test should be considered. On the other hand, in a population at low risk of trisomy 21, failure to visualize the fetal nasal bone could easily be a variation of normal.

Bibliography

1. Cicero S, Curcio P, Papageorghiou A, Sonek J, Nicolaides K. Absence of nasal bone in fetuses with trisomy 21 at 11–14 weeks of gestation: an observational study. Lancet 2001; 358(9294): 1665–7.
2. Prefumo F, Sairam S, Bhide A, Thilaganathan B. First-trimester nuchal translucency, nasal bones, and trisomy 21 in selected and unselected populations. Am J Obstet Gynecol 2006; 194(3): 828–33.

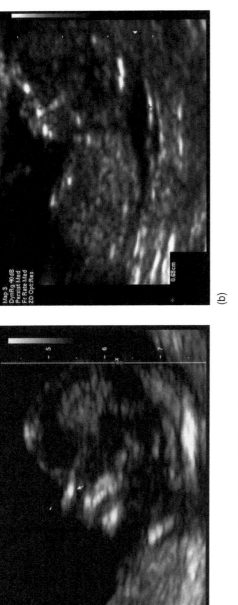

(a)

(b)

Fig. 5.1 *(a) First trimester nasal bones (b) First trimester absent nasal bones*

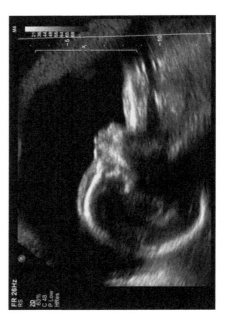

Fig. 5.2 *Second trimester hypoplastic nasal bone*

6

MICROGNATHIA

The chin is best visualized on a mid-sagittal profile view of the face. There is no definition for micrognathia, and the diagnosis is subjective. Unless micrognathia is severe, ultrasound diagnosis is extremely difficult. Even when a diagnosis of micrognathia is made, it may be an isolated finding which resolves with advancing pregnancy or with conservative management in the infant period.

Trisomies 13 and 18

A careful examination should be conducted to exclude other markers of trisomy 18 (choroid plexus cysts, ventriculomegaly, clenched fists, congenital heart disease, congenital diaphragmatic hernia, exomphalos, single umbilical artery, and talipes) or trisomy 13 (holoprosencephaly, congenital heart disease, and polydactyly).

Goldenhar syndrome

This is also known as 'hemifacial microsomia'. There is asymmetry between structures on the left/right sides of the face. In addition to craniofacial anomalies, there may be cardiac, vertebral, and central nervous system defects. Most cases are sporadic, but some show autosomal dominant inheritance.

Other genetic syndromes

Many genetic syndromes can be associated with the finding of micrognathia. They include DiGeorge, Treacher Collins, Pierre Robin, and Smith–Lemli–Opitz syndromes. Typically, ultrasound prenatal diagnosis is difficult in these syndromes, as the majority of associated features are not seen on ultrasound or are diagnosed late in pregnancy.

Bibliography

1. Bromley B, Benacerraf BR. Fetal micrognathia: associated anomalies and outcome. J Ultrasound Med 1994; 13(7): 529–33.
2. Rotten D, Levaillant JM, Martinez H, Ducou le Pointe H, Vicaut E. The fetal mandible: a 2D and 3D sonographic approach to the diagnosis of retrognathia and micrognathia. Ultrasound Obstet Gynecol 2002; 19(2): 122–30.

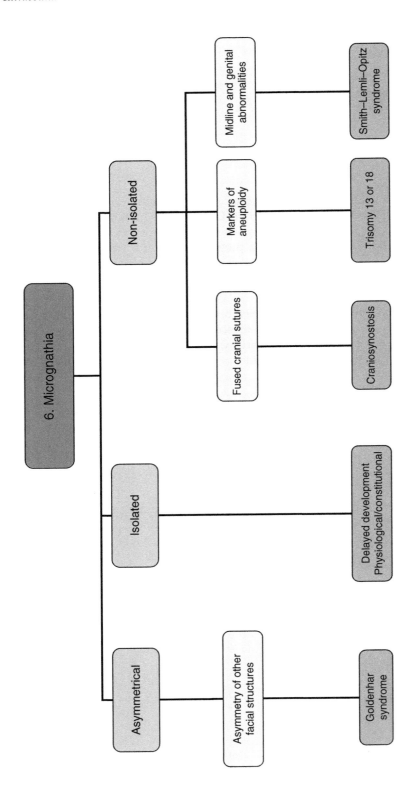

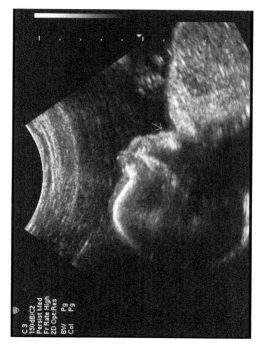

Fig. 6.1 *Micrognathia*

7

CHEST TUMOURS

The majority of fetal chest tumours are benign and tend to be identified in the second trimester. In the absence of fetal hydrops, they usually have a favourable prognosis. The vast majority of chest lesions tend to be unilateral, possibly because bilateral lesions are self-limiting. In many cases they present with mediastinal shift, easily spotted, with the heart axis being deviated to one side (see 'Dextrocardia').

Congenital cystic adenomatoid malformation

These lesions may be unilateral/bilateral and microcystic/macrocystic. Bilateral lesions may cause hydrops and fetal demise as a consequence of cardiac compression.

Pulmonary sequestration

The presence of systemic arterial supply from the thoracic or abdominal dorsal aorta would be characteristic of pulmonary sequestration. These benign tumours may cause hyperdynamic heart failure and hydrops as a consequence of an arterio-venous bypass effect.

Bronchial obstruction

The appearance is similar to a microcystic congenital cystic adenomatoid malformation (CCAM), but typically the diaphragmatic domes are not flattened. Resolution usually occurs in a matter of a few weeks, as opposed to months in the case of CCAM.

Congenital diaphragmatic hernia

The presence of a unilateral lesion with mixed echoes should raise the suspicion of a congenital diaphragmatic hernia (CDH), especially with mediastinal deviation and the lack of a stomach bubble in the normal position.

Congenital high airway obstruction syndrome

The presence of bilateral chest lesions suggests either bilateral CCAM or congenital high airway obstruction syndrome (CHAOS). The latter usually has the additional feature of dilated airways. A significant proportion also present with ascites owing to obstruction to the venous return to the heart.

Midline chest lesions

Midline chest lesions are very rare and may be of enteric, thymic, or pericardial origin. Enteric or bronchogenic midline tumours are usually cystic and tend to be benign. Pericardial tumours are usually teratomas and may present initially as pericardial effusions. Depending on their exact site on the pericardial surface, they may cause rhythm disturbances.

Bibliography

1. Geary MP, Chitty LS, Morrison JJ et al. Perinatal outcome and prognostic factors in prenatally diagnosed congenital diaphragmatic hernia. Ultrasound Obstet Gynecol 1998; 12(2): 107–11.
2. Ierullo AM, Ganapathy R, Crowley S et al. Neonatal outcome of antenatally diagnosed congenital cystic adenomatoid malformations. Ultrasound Obstet Gynecol 2005; 26(2): 150–3.

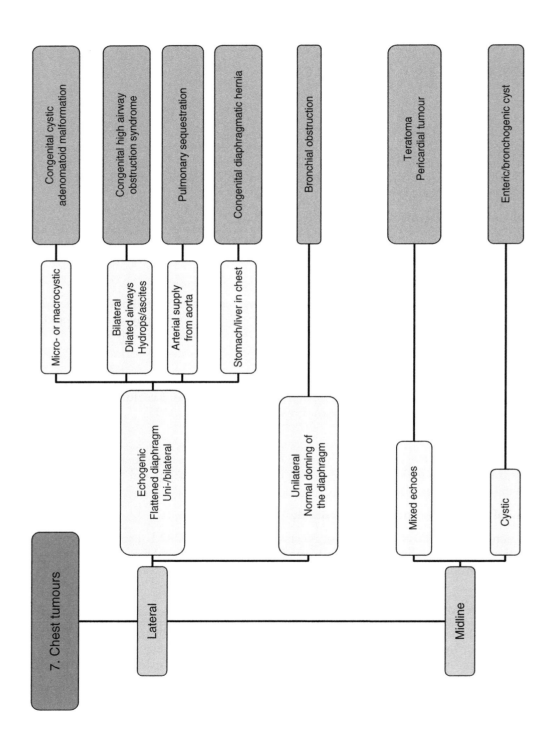

7. Chest tumours

Lateral

Echogenic
Flattened diaphragm
Uni-/bilateral

Micro- or macrocystic — Congenital cystic adenomatoid malformation

Bilateral
Dilated airways
Hydrops/ascites — Congenital high airway obstruction syndrome

Arterial supply from aorta — Pulmonary sequestration

Stomach/liver in chest — Congenital diaphragmatic hernia

Unilateral
Normal doming of the diaphragm — Bronchial obstruction

Midline

Mixed echoes — Teratoma
Pericardial tumour

Cystic — Enteric/bronchogenic cyst

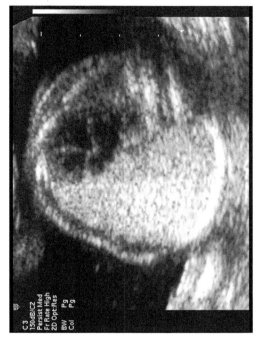

Fig. 7.2 *Microcystic lung lesion*

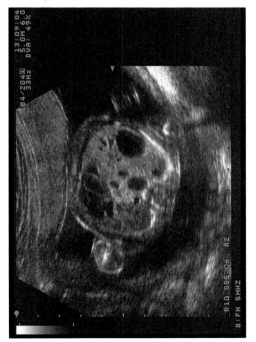

Fig. 7.1 *Macrocystic lung lesion*

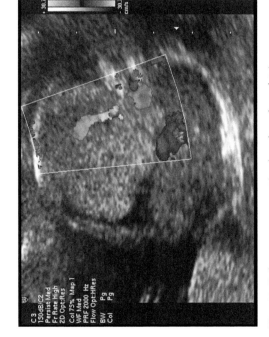

Fig. 7.3 *Pulmonary sequestration (see also colour plate)*

8

CHEST FLUID

Fluid in the fetal chest is seen relatively commonly either as a cystic collection or as pleural or pericardial effusion. Cystic collections in the lungs or mediastinum need to be dealt with as chest tumours. Pleural effusion is seen as fluid collection around the compressed lung. Pleural or pericardial effusions may occur simultaneously in some conditions, but usually tend to be independent of each other.

Pleural effusion

This is usually present as part of a fetal hydrops, accompanying a structural anomaly, or, more rarely, an isolated finding. Most primary pleural effusions occur due to either excessive production or reduced reabsorption of lymphatic fluid. Complex or secondary pleural effusions may result from aneuploidy, congenital viral infection, fetal anaemia (usually with skin oedema), and hyperdynamic cardiac failure from arterio-venous shunting (with vascular tumours such as placental chorioangioma). Even in the absence of any other chromosomal marker, pleural effusion carries a 10% risk for chromosomal abnormalities.

Pericardial effusion

Prenatal sonographic identification of a small rim of pericardial fluid is a normal finding. Pericardial effusion is a subjective diagnosis, unless the fluid collection is obviously large. It may be an isolated finding or result from an underlying pericardial tumour or fetal arrhythmia/cardiac structural abnormality, or rarely it may be found with a cardiac aneurysm/diverticulum.

Bibliography

1. Santolaya-Forgas J. How do we counsel patients carrying a fetus with pleural effusions? Ultrasound Obstet Gynecol 2001; 18(4): 305–8.
2. Slesnick TC, Ayres NA, Altman CA et al. Characteristics and outcomes of fetuses with pericardial effusions. Am J Cardiol 2005; 96(4): 599–601.

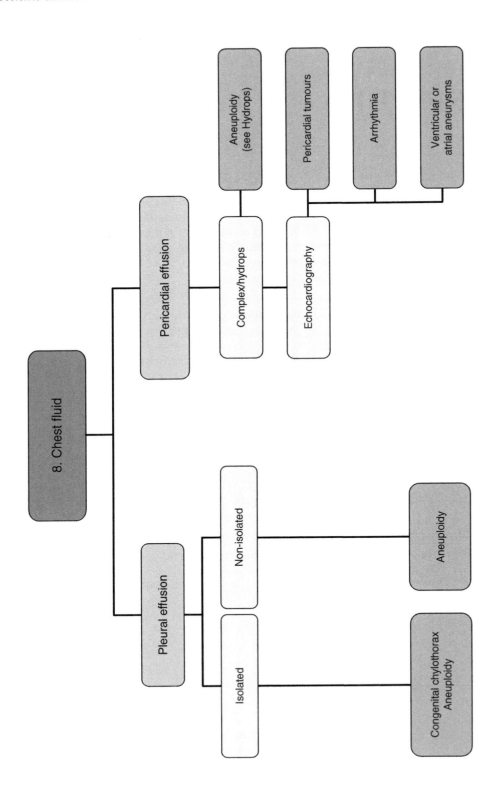

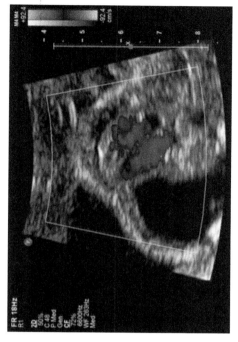

Fig. 8.1 *Mild pleural effusion*

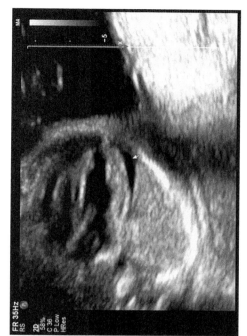

Fig. 8.2 *Moderate pleural effusion & mediastinal shift (see also colour plate)*

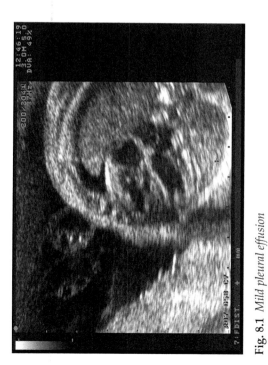

Fig. 8.3 *Severe pleural effusion & fetal hydrops*

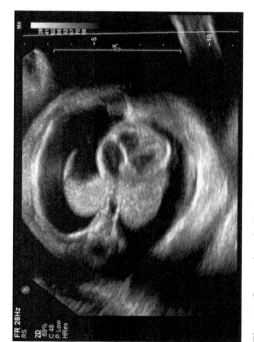

Fig. 8.4 *Pericardial effusion*

9

DEXTROCARDIA

Fetal dextrocardia is a condition in which the major axis of the heart (from the base to the apex along the interventricular septum) points to the right. The term dextrocardia describes only the position of the cardiac axis and conveys no information regarding chamber organization and structural anatomy of the heart. Dextrocardia should be distinguished from dextroposition, in which the heart is shifted into the right chest as a consequence of pathological states involving the diaphragm, lung, pleura, or other adjoining tissues.

Dextroposition

The commonest cause of dextroposition is the presence of chest fluid or a tumour (see previous chapters). In the absence of such space occupying lesions, consideration should be given to the diagnosis of scimitar syndrome: a smaller right side in the fetal chest with hypoplasia of the right lung and anomalous pulmonary venous drainage.

Dextrocardia

True dextrocardia tends to be associated with situs abnormalities. Situs by definition relates to the fetal left–right orientation of chest and abdominal organs. Situs can be assessed at various levels, namely abdominal, atrial, and pulmonary levels, and is usually similar at all levels. Situs solitus refers to the usual (normal) arrangement of left and right sided structures with the dorsal aorta in the left side of the fetal abdomen and the inferior vena cava (IVC) on the right. With true dextrocardia, the likelihood of structural cardiac abnormalities increases, especially of cardiac isomerisms. In the presence of situs inversus and dextrocardia with a structurally normal heart, the child will still need postnatal follow-up for other associated conditions such as Kartagener syndrome (ciliary dyskinesia).

Bibliography

1. Bernasconi A, Azancot A, Simpson JM, Jones A, Sharland GK. Fetal dextrocardia: diagnosis and outcome in two tertiary centres. Heart 2005; 91(12): 1590–4.
2. Holzmann D, Ott PM, Felix H. Diagnostic approach to primary ciliary dyskinesia: a review. Eur J Pediatr 2000; 159(1–2): 95–8.

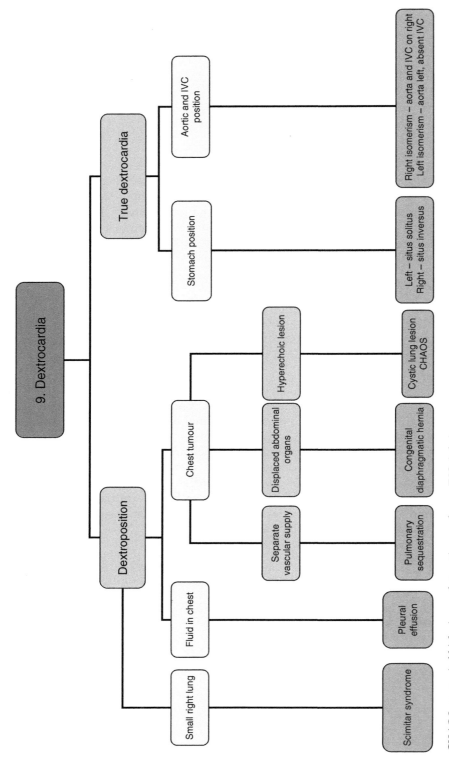

CHAOS, congenital high airway obstruction syndrome; IVC, inferior vena cava.

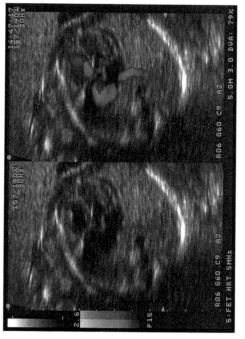

Fig. 9.2 *Dextrocardia (see also colour plate)*

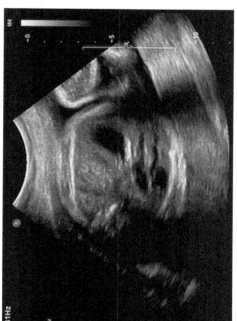

Fig. 9.1 *Congenital diaphragmatic hernia*

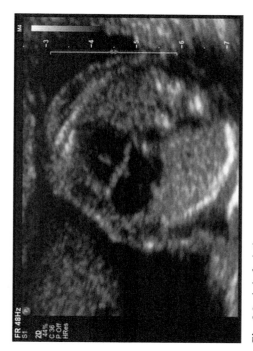

Fig. 9.3 *Axis deviation*

10

ABNORMAL FOUR-CHAMBER VIEW

It is important to consider what should be routinely examined while checking a fetal heart:

1. Check abdominal situs. First confirm the left and right of the fetus and ensure that the fetal heart and stomach are on the fetal left side.
2. Check that the fetal heart points to the left with the majority of the heart in the left chest.
3. Check that the heart occupies a third of the chest area.
4. Check that there are four chambers with symmetrical ventricles and atria.
5. Ensure that the moderator band is identified and indicates the right ventricle.
6. Check that there are two atrio-ventricular valves opening and closing (cineloop helps) and that their point of attachment to the interventricular septum shows an offset, with the tricuspid valve being closer to the apex when compared to the mitral valve.
7. Check that the septum is intact (preferably examined with the septum horizontally oriented).
8. Further examinations should check the outflow tracts and ensure crossover. Much of this can be assessed using the three-vessel view.

Cardiomegaly

This finding should prompt assessment of the haemodynamic state in the fetus. It is usually secondary to some other fetal pathology including growth restriction, hyperdynamic circulatory states such as anaemia, arterio-venous malformations in the fetus, placental chorioangioma, and occasionally fetal brady- or tachyarrhythmias. Primary causes include major cardiac structural abnormalities, and will need detailed assessment that is beyond the scope of this chapter.

Asymmetry of the cardiac chambers

This usually reflects a structural problem in the atrio-ventricular or outflow tract valves. Rare causes include anomalous venous drainage of the pulmonary veins, where the drainage is into the right side of the heart rather than the left side of the heart in one or more veins.

Loss of the atrio-ventricular valve offset

The loss of a normal offset between the atrio-ventricular valves suggests the presence of an atrio-ventricular canal defect called the atrio-ventricular septal defect. This is associated with a 50–60% risk of chromosomal abnormality. A significant proportion of these cases will also have situs abnormalities (see chapter on 'Dextrocardia').

Bibliography

1. Bolnick AD, Zelop CM, Milewski B et al. Use of the mitral valve-tricuspid valve distance as a marker of fetal endocardial cushion defects. Am J Obstet Gynecol 2004; 191(4): 1483–5.
2. Del Bianco A, Russo S, Lacerenza N et al. Four chamber view plus three-vessel and trachea view for a complete evaluation of the fetal heart during the second trimester. J Perinat Med 2006; 34(4): 309–12.
3. Vergani P, Mariani S, Ghidini A et al. Screening for congenital heart disease with the four-chamber view of the fetal heart. Am J Obstet Gynecol 1992; 167(4 Pt 1): 1000–3.

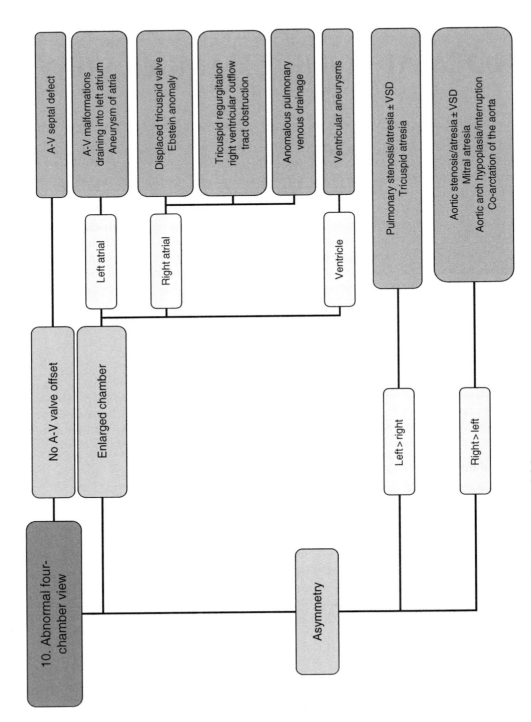

A-V, atrio-ventricular; VSD, ventricular septal defect.

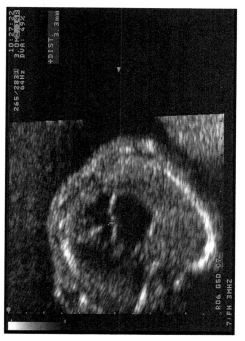

Fig. 10.1 *Ventricular asymmetry*

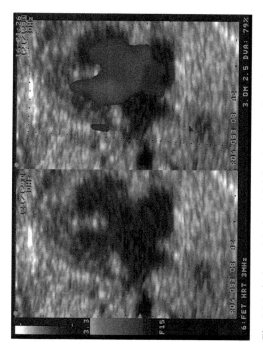

Fig. 10.2 *Ventricular septal defect*

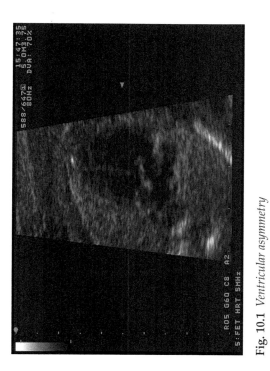

Fig. 10.3 *Colour Doppler demonstration of ventriculoseptal defect*

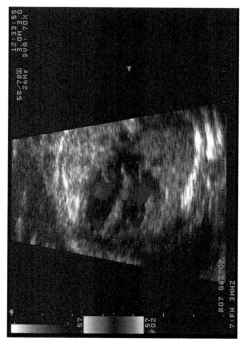

Fig. 10.4 *Atrio-ventriculoseptal defect (see also colour plate)*

11

ANTERIOR ABDOMINAL WALL DEFECT

The physiological gut herniation into the umbilical sac is restored to the normal position by approximately 10–11 weeks. Any abnormality after 11 weeks needs to be assessed carefully.

Exomphalos

The presence of a sac at the umbilicus with gut or liver contained in it is likely to be an exomphalos. The umbilical cord vessels can be seen traversing through this sac, which can vary in size. There is a strong association with chromosomal abnormality.

Bladder and cloacal extrophy

If the defect extends infra-umbilically, it is likely to involve the fetal bladder (non-visualized bladder) and possibly the genitalia (ambiguous genitalia). Under these circumstances, postnatal surgery is likely to involve reconstruction of the external genitalia and possibly gender re-assignment in some fetuses.

Beckwith–Wiedemann syndrome

If the exomphalos is small with features of macrosomia and organomegaly in the fetus, a diagnosis of Beckwith–Wiedemann syndrome can be made, and has implications for follow-up apart from surgery.

Pentalogy of Cantrell

If the anterior wall defect is more extensive superior to the umbilicus, it might involve parts of the diaphragm, pericardium, and the fetal heart as part of the pentalogy of Cantrell.

Body stalk anomaly

In some cases, a sac with the intra-abdominal contents is seen along with distortion of the spinal cord, poorly developed lower limbs, and a very short umbilical cord. These features form part of the body stalk anomaly or amniotic rupture sequence, and are uniformly associated with very poor prognosis.

Gastroschisis

The bowel is seen herniated without a sac (cauliflower-like appearance), just lateral to the cord insertion. Gastroschisis is usually located to the right of the umbilical cord, which has a normal insertion. The herniated organs usually only include loops of bowel, and there is no association with chromosomal abnormality.

Bibliography

1. Barisic I, Clementi M, Hausler M et al. Euroscan Study Group. Evaluation of prenatal ultrasound diagnosis of fetal abdominal wall defects by 19 European registries. Ultrasound Obstet Gynecol 2001; 18(4): 309–16.
2. Smrcek JM, Germer U, Krokowski M et al. Prenatal ultrasound diagnosis and management of body stalk anomaly: analysis of nine singleton and two multiple pregnancies. Ultrasound Obstet Gynecol 2003; 21(4): 322–8.
3. Williams DH, Gauthier DW, Maizels M. Prenatal diagnosis of Beckwith-Wiedemann syndrome. Prenat Diagn 2005; 25(10): 879–84.

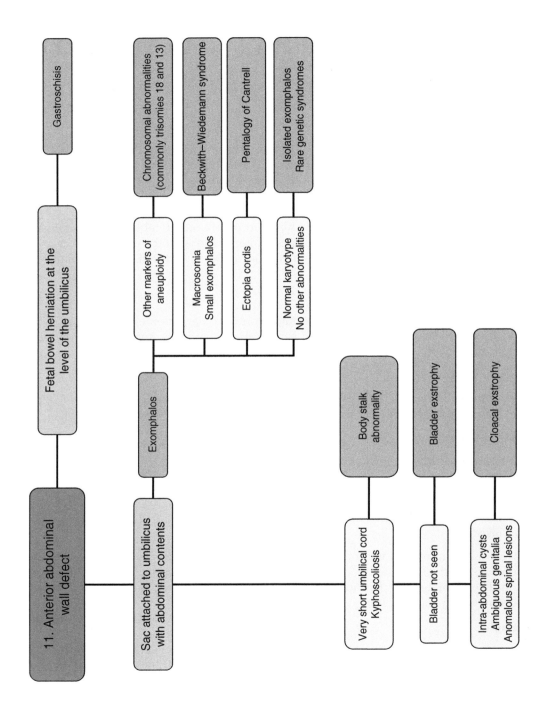

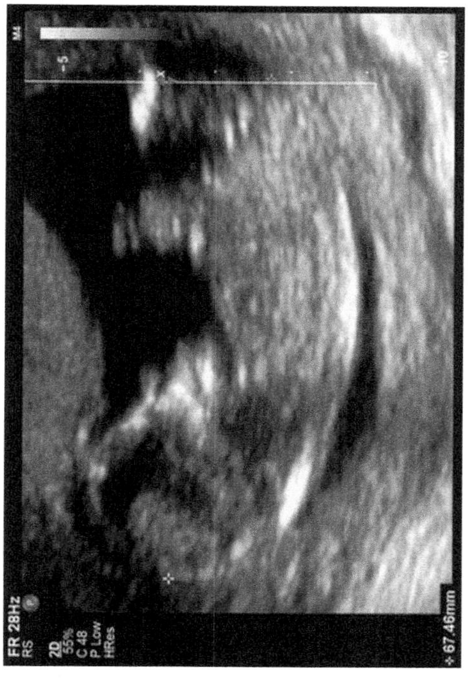

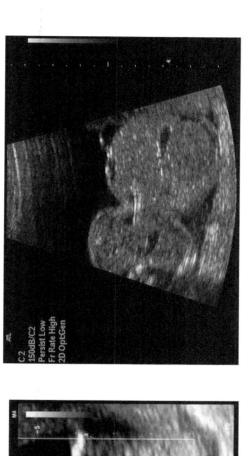

Fig. 11.2 *Large exomphalos*

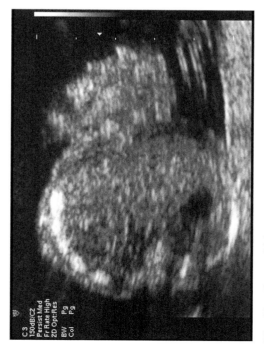

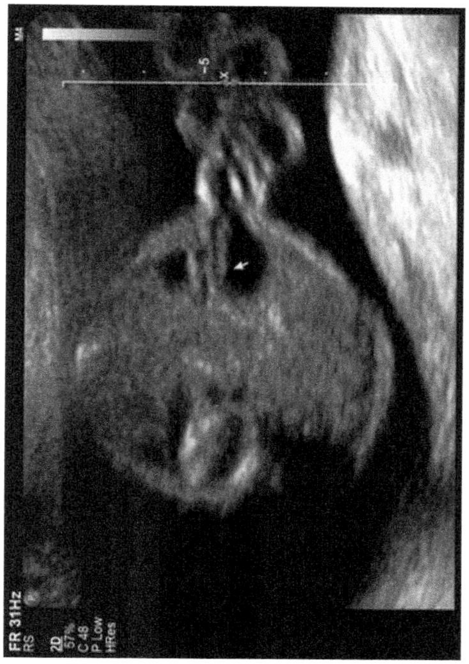

Fig. 11.4 *Umbilical cord cyst*

Fig. 11.1 *First trimester exomphalos*

Fig. 11.3 *Gastroschisis*

12

ABDOMINAL CYSTS

Cystic lesions in the fetal abdomen present as either isolated or multiple anechoic areas. The correct diagnosis of these is difficult antenatally and most cysts remain indeterminate in origin. The outcome is usually dependent on the site and origin of these cysts and the presence of any associated abnormalities.

Isolated cystic lesions

Isolated cystic lesions are quite common and are usually considered benign. Their relationship to the fetal bladder is important in determining their origin. A cystic lesion supero-lateral to the fetal bladder (frequently bilateral with septations) is suggestive of an ovarian cyst in a female fetus. In fetuses of either sex, the differential diagnosis would include mesenteric and intestinal duplication cysts. Anterior meningoceles and hydrometrocolpos (female fetus) are seen as cysts posterior to the fetal bladder. Rarely, the cyst may be seen totally unrelated to the bladder and in the upper abdomen. If this is on the right, one should consider a benign liver cyst if the gall bladder is visualized and appears normal. The non-visualization of the gall bladder suggests a choledochal cyst.

Multiple cystic urogenital lesions

Multiple lesions are usually related to either the fetal bowel or fetal kidneys. The presence of hydronephrosis with a dilated, convoluted fluid-filled (echo-free) structure connecting the kidney to the bladder is diagnostic of mega-ureter. The latter usually results from either vesico-ureteric reflux or vesico-ureteric junction obstruction. The presence of a dilated bladder with bilateral mega-ureters is diagnostic of bladder outlet obstruction.

Multiple cystic bowel lesions

Typically, bowel obstruction manifests in the third trimester with multiple linear or discrete cystic spaces that connect with one another. Additionally they have internal echoes that give a speckled appearance. A double bubble appearance in the fetal upper abdomen is suggestive of a high small intestinal obstruction with a high risk for chromosomal abnormality. The exact site(s) or cause (intrinsic: atresia, web; extrinsic: volvulus, peritoneal bands) of the obstruction(s) is not detectable antenatally. Additional features such as echogenic bowel or ascitic fluid collection indicate the possibility of meconium peritonitis which is more common in cystic fibrosis.

Dilatation of the large bowel also manifests in the third trimester, but is usually not detectable on ultrasound.

Bibliography

1. Casaccia G, Bilancioni E, Nahom A et al. Cystic anomalies of biliary tree in the fetus: is it possible to make a more specific prenatal diagnosis? J Pediatr Surg 2002; 37(8): 1191–4.
2. Heling KS, Chaoui R, Kirchmair F, Stadie S, Bollmann R. Fetal ovarian cysts: prenatal diagnosis, management and postnatal outcome. Ultrasound Obstet Gynecol 2002; 20(1): 47–50.
3. McEwing R, Hayward C, Furness M. Foetal cystic abdominal masses. Australas Radiol 2003; 47(2): 101–10.

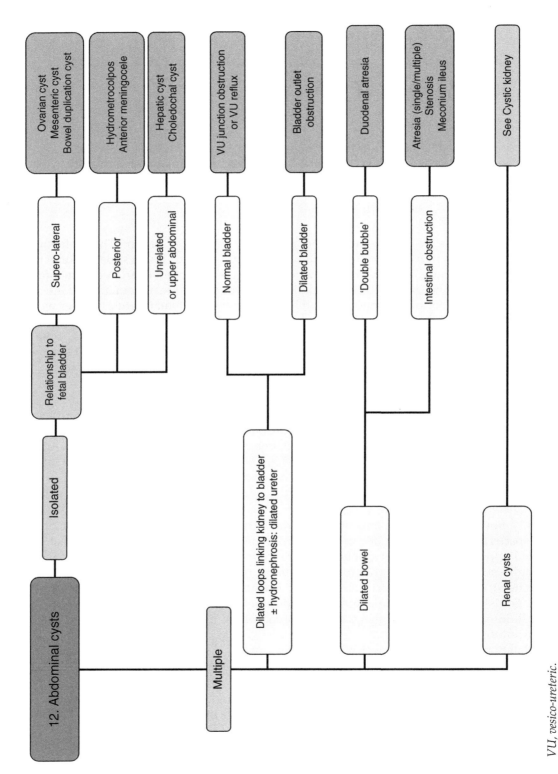

VU, vesico-ureteric.

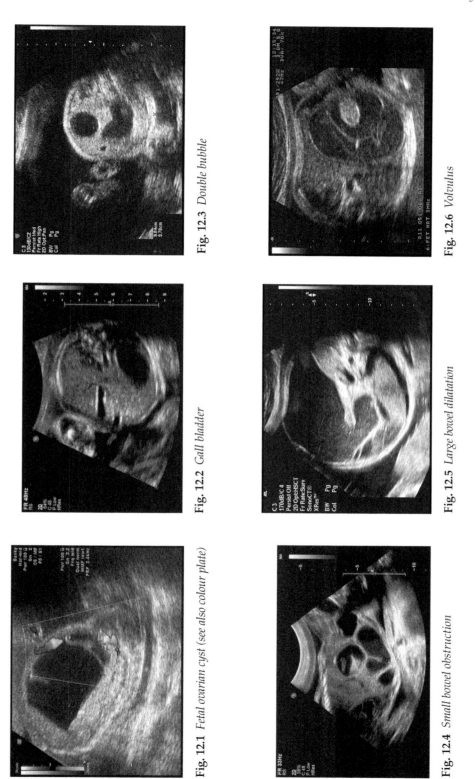

Fig. 12.1 *Fetal ovarian cyst (see also colour plate)*

Fig. 12.2 *Gall bladder*

Fig. 12.3 *Double bubble*

Fig. 12.4 *Small bowel obstruction*

Fig. 12.5 *Large bowel dilatation*

Fig. 12.6 *Volvulus*

13

ABDOMINAL ECHOGENICITY

The finding of increased echogenicity in the fetal abdomen is common. These hyperechoic areas may be in the fetal bowel, kidneys, or the liver.

Hyperechoic kidneys

Echogenic kidneys in the presence of dilated renal outflow tracts are suggestive of poor function in the kidneys. If the liquor volume is normal, then this is likely to be a normal variant with a normal neonatal outcome. The presence of reduced liquor volume with bright kidneys suggests renal failure, and is likely to be associated with a poor outcome. Infantile polycystic kidneys usually manifest as large bright kidneys without any cortico-medullary differentiation. This invariably presents with anhydramnios and is a lethal malformation.

Hyperechoic bowel

This is the most common echogenic mass in the fetal abdomen. By definition the bowel is considered echogenic only if it is as bright as or brighter than the adjacent bone, namely, the iliac crest. The commonest cause for echogenic bowel is fetal ingestion of blood. This is usually identified as 'floating flakes' in the amniotic fluid and is invariably associated with a history of vaginal bleeding. As an isolated finding, it would not increase the risk for chromosomal abnormalities. The presence of associated bowel dilatation with or without ascitic fluid should raise the possibility of meconium ileus, which is more common with cystic fibrosis.

Discrete hyperechoic foci

Discrete echogenic foci in the fetal abdomen are a common finding at the routine anomaly scan, and are generally associated with a good outcome. The presence of other foci seen in other organs (brain, chest, etc.) is suggestive of congenital viral infection.

Bibliography

1. McNamara A, Levine D. Intra-abdominal fetal echogenic masses: a practical guide to diagnosis and management. Radiographics 2005; 25(3): 633–45.
2. Sepulveda W, Leung KY, Robertson ME et al. Prevalence of cystic fibrosis mutations in pregnancies with fetal echogenic bowel. Obstet Gynecol 1996; 87(1): 103–6.
3. Simchen MJ, Toi A, Bona M et al. Fetal hepatic calcifications: prenatal diagnosis and outcome. Am J Obstet Gynecol 2002; 187(6): 1617–22.

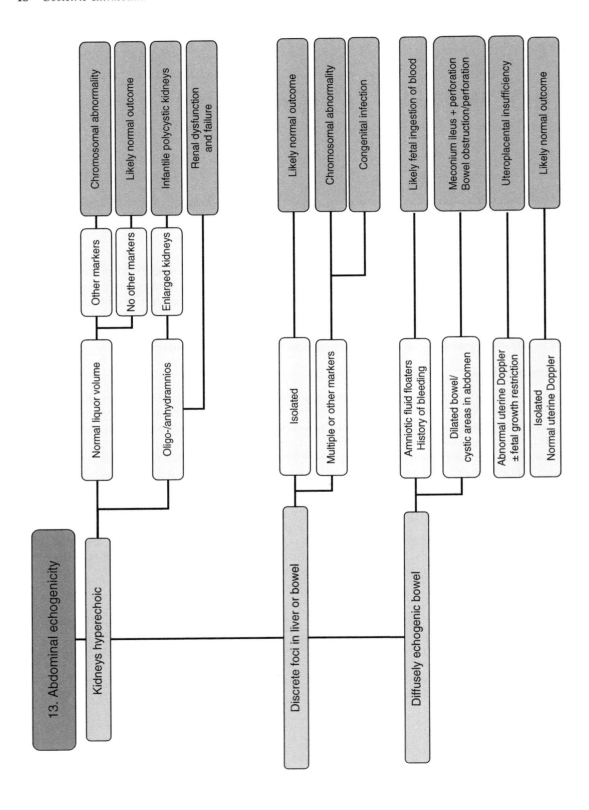

13. Abdominal echogenicity

Kidneys hyperechoic
- Normal liquor volume
  - Other markers → Chromosomal abnormality
  - No other markers → Likely normal outcome
- Oligo-/anhydramnios
  - Enlarged kidneys → Infantile polycystic kidneys
  - Renal dysfunction and failure

Discrete foci in liver or bowel
- Isolated → Likely normal outcome
- Multiple or other markers → Chromosomal abnormality
- Congenital infection

Diffusely echogenic bowel
- Amniotic fluid floaters / History of bleeding → Likely fetal ingestion of blood
- Dilated bowel/cystic areas in abdomen → Meconium ileus + perforation / Bowel obstruction/perforation
- Abnormal uterine Doppler ± fetal growth restriction → Uteroplacental insufficiency
- Isolated / Normal uterine Doppler → Likely normal outcome

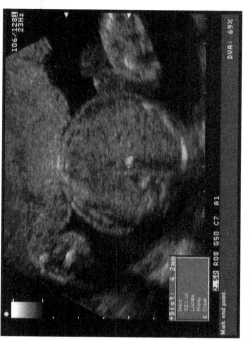

Fig. 13.2 *Echogenic focus in liver*

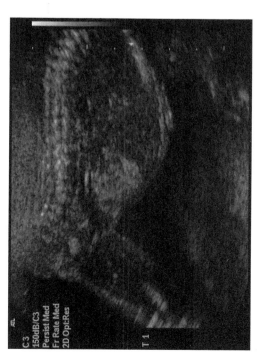

Fig. 13.1 *Hyperechogenic bowel*

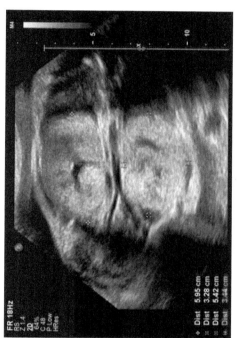

Fig. 13.3 *Hyperechogenic kidneys*

14

EMPTY RENAL FOSSA

In fetal life the normal kidneys are imaged with ease in the renal fossae from about 16 weeks of gestation.

Agenesis or ectopic kidney?

Absence of renal tissue in the normal site, namely the renal fossa, may be due to true agenesis or to ectopic presentation of the kidney. The latter could be either in the fetal pelvis or due to a fusion with the contralateral kidney. In either case, the kidney could show signs of pelvicalyceal dilatation due to the abnormal position and contour of the drainage system. In true agenesis, the renal artery is absent on the ipsilateral side. Ectopic kidneys derive their blood supply from the aorta or the iliac arteries. Unilateral agenesis is usually an isolated finding, but may be part of the VACTERL association (vertebral, anal, cardiac, tracheo-(o)esophageal, (o)esophageal, renal, or limb abnormalities).

Bilateral renal agenesis

Bilateral renal agenesis is usually a diagnosis of exclusion, with the presentation being that of anhydramnios in the second trimester. The renal fossae are hard to image due to the lack of liquor. Additionally, the suprarenal glands occupy the renal fossae, mimicking normal renal tissue on scan. The lack of a normally filled bladder and renal arteries in the setting of anhydramnios would be features in favour of bilateral renal agenesis.

Bibliography

1. Bhide A, Sairam S, Farrugia MK, Boddy SA, Thilaganathan B. The sensitivity of antenatal ultrasound for predicting renal tract surgery in early childhood. Ultrasound Obstet Gynecol 2005; 25(5): 489–92.
2. Sepulveda W, Stagiannis KD, Flack NJ, Fisk NM. Accuracy of prenatal diagnosis of renal agenesis with color flow imaging in severe second-trimester oligohydramnios. Am J Obstet Gynecol 1995; 173(6): 1788–92.

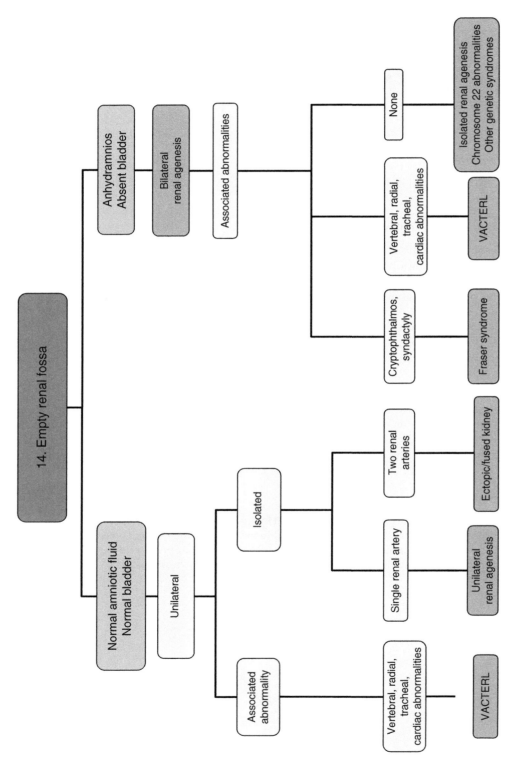

VACTERL, vertebral, anal, cardiac, tracheo-(o)esophageal, (o)esophageal, renal, limb.

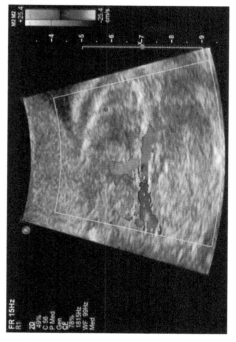

Fig. 14.1 *Unilateral renal agenesis*

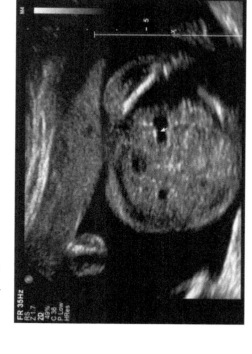

Fig. 14.2 *Single renal artery in unilateral renal agenesis (see also colour plate)*

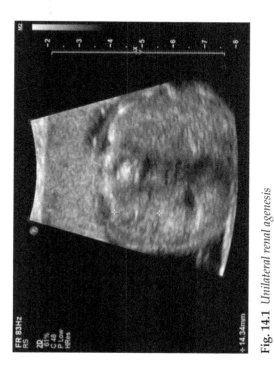

Fig. 14.3 *Absent renal arteries in bilateral renal agenesis (see also colour plate)*

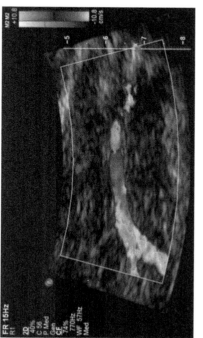

Fig. 14.4 *Pelvic kidney*

15

CYSTIC KIDNEY

Cystic kidney is a common finding in routine antenatal screening. As a general rule, regardless of the diagnosis, the presence of a normal amniotic fluid volume is indicative of a good prognosis. The finding of anhydramnios in the presence of renal abnormalities would confer a poor prognosis from either pulmonary hypoplasia or renal failure.

Solitary cyst

Solitary cysts in the renal cortex in one or both kidneys may be an isolated finding, but should raise the possibility of adult polycystic disease. In some, there might be demonstrable cysts in the fetal liver and spleen. The bladder and liquor volume are usually normal in this situation. As this is a dominant disorder, the parents should have renal scans.

Isolated multiple cysts

Multiple cysts with a dysplastic kidney can be unilateral (usually normal amniotic fluid volume) or bilateral (usually anhydramnios). There is no clear differentiation between cortex and medulla, with the cysts being randomly distributed, distorting the renal outline. Unilateral multicystic dysplastic kidney has a very good prognosis, provided that the contralateral kidney and amniotic fluid volume are normal.

Multiple cysts with associated findings

Bilateral multicystic kidneys are usually associated with anhydramnios or severe oligohydramnios, and this interferes with the assessment of the rest of the fetal anatomy. However, the identification of macrosomia with a small exomphalos would suggest Beckwith–Wiedemann syndrome. Multisystem abnormalities such as vertebral and cardiac anomalies would favour a diagnosis of VATER (vertebral, anal, tracheo-(o)esophageal, (o)esophageal, renal) or VACTERL (as above, plus cardiac, limb) associations or chromosomal abnormalities such as trisomy 13 or 18. The presence of polydactyly along with an encephalocele would strongly suggest the possibility of the autosomal recessive Meckel–Gruber syndrome. A number of genetic syndromes are diagnosed after a postnatal assessment of the baby or after a post-mortem examination.

Bibliography

1. Lazebnik N, Bellinger MF, Ferguson JE 2nd, Hogge JS, Hogge WA. Insights into the pathogenesis and natural history of fetuses with multicystic dysplastic kidney disease. Prenat Diagn 1999; 19(5): 418–23.
2. van Eijk L, Cohen-Overbeek TE, den Hollander NS, Nijman JM, Wladimiroff JW. Unilateral multicystic dysplastic kidney: a combined pre- and postnatal assessment. Ultrasound Obstet Gynecol 2002; 19(2): 180–3.

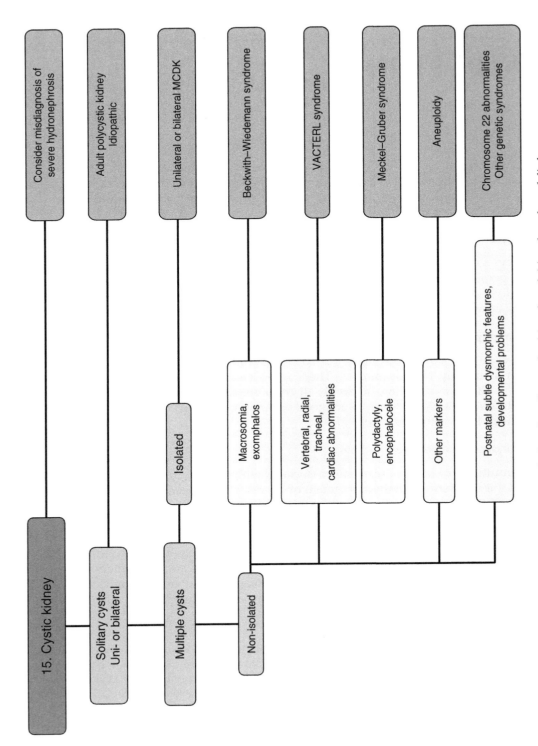

MCDK, multicystic dysplastic kidney; VACTERL, vertebral, anal, cardiac, tracheo-(o)esophageal, (o)esophageal, renal, limb.

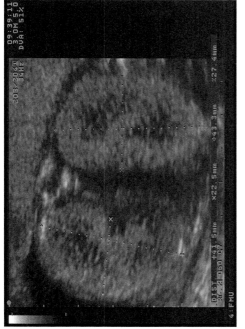

Fig. 15.2 *Infantile polycystic kidney*

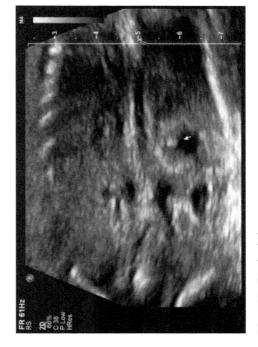

Fig. 15.3 *Duplex kidney*

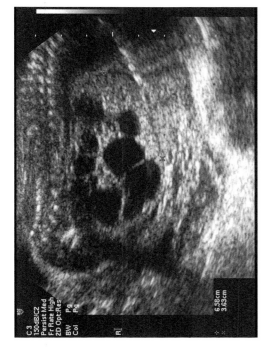

Fig. 15.1 *Multicystic kidney*

16

FLUID FILLED KIDNEY

Renal pelvis dilatation (hydronephrosis or pyelectasia) is present in approximately 2–3% of all fetuses in mid-gestation. Hydronephrosis is considered to be mild if the antero-posterior dimension of the renal pelvis is 4–7 mm in the absence of calyceal dilatation. Hydronephrosis is classified as moderate/severe if the renal pelvis antero-posterior measurement is over 7 mm or if there is calyceal dilatation.

Risk of chromosomal abnormality

The presence of hydronephrosis should prompt a thorough search for other soft markers for chromosomal abnormalities. In isolation, hydronephrosis does not increase the risk for chromosomal anomalies. The presence of any additional anomalies would significantly increase the background risk of a chromosomal abnormality.

Natural history

The majority of mild hydronephrosis cases (> 85%) tend to resolve spontaneously, with the remainder only requiring postnatal investigations. Persistent hydronephrosis is defined as a renal pelvis antero-posterior diameter of > 10 mm at > 28 weeks, and suggests the possibility of pelvi-ureteric junction obstruction, or vesico-ureteric junction obstruction or reflux (typically bilateral). With persistent third trimester hydronephrosis, approximately 1 in 3 babies will need postnatal corrective surgery. The presence of ureteric dilatation (vesico-ureteric obstruction or vesico-ureteric reflux) should be noted, as the neonate will need prophylactic antibiotics.

Bibliography

1. Livera LN, Brookfield DSK, Egginton JA, Hawnaur JM. Antenatal ultrasonography to detect fetal abnormalities: a prospective screening programme. BMJ 1989; 298(6685): 1421–3.
2. Sairam S, Al-Habib A, Sasson S, Thilaganathan B. Natural history of fetal hydronephrosis diagnosed on mid-trimester ultrasound. Ultrasound Obstet Gynecol 2001; 17(3): 191–6.
3. Thompson MO, Thilaganathan B. Effect of routine screening for Down's syndrome on the significance of isolated fetal hydronephrosis. Br J Obstet Gynaecol 1998; 105(8): 860–4.

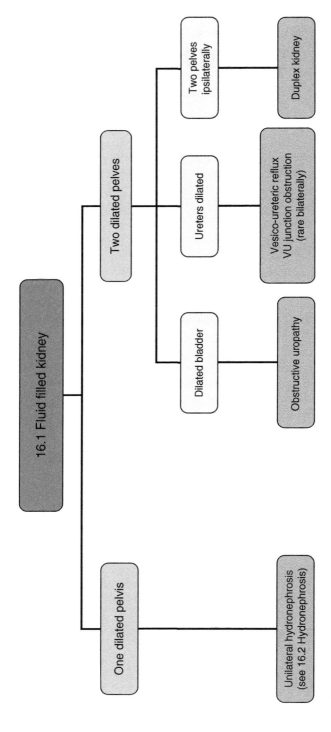

VU, vesico-ureteric.

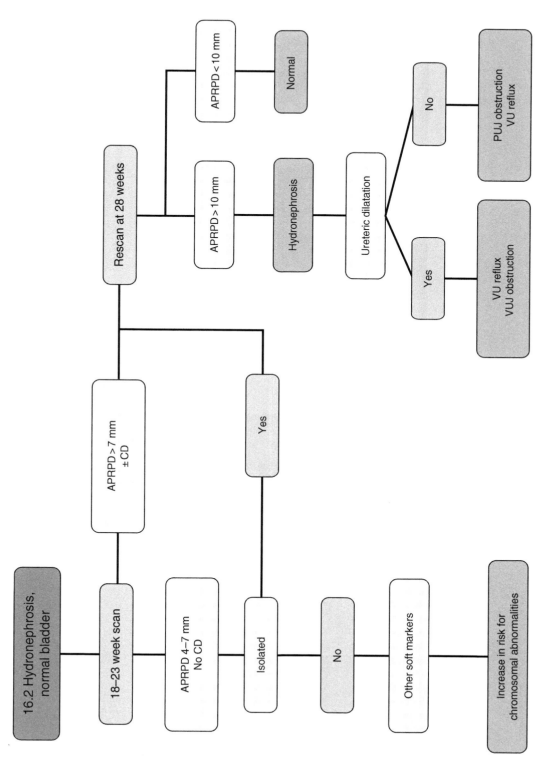

APRPD, antero-posterior renal pelvis diameter; CD, calyceal dilatation; VU, vesico-ureteric; VUJ, vesico-ureteric junction; PUJ, pelvi-ureteric junction.

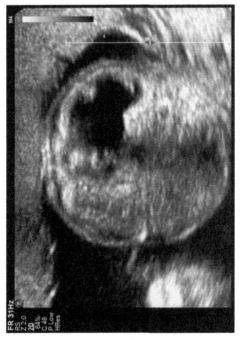

Fig. 16.2 *Severe hydronephrosis*

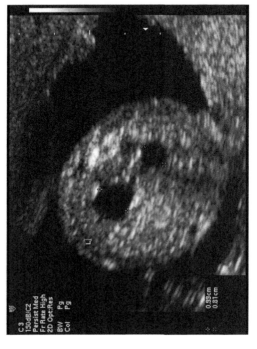

Fig. 16.1 *Moderate hydronephrosis*

17

ABNORMAL BLADDER

The fetal bladder can be easily visualized in all stages of pregnancy. The bladder should always be assessed in combination with the liquor volume and the kidneys.

Megacystis

In the first trimester, an enlarged bladder > 7 mm (megacystis) should raise the suspicion of either chromosomal abnormalities or obstructive uropathy. Approximately 20% of fetuses with megacystis measuring 7–15 mm have an underlying chromosomal abnormality such as trisomy 13 or 18. If the bladder measures > 15 mm, the risk of an underlying bladder outlet obstruction (urethral atresia, posterior urethral valves, or cloacal abnormalities) is very high and is associated with a very poor prognosis. With megacystis > 15 mm, it is sometimes possible to find echogenic or dysplastic kidneys and reduced liquor volume in the first trimester.

Intermittent/partial urethral obstruction

The finding of an enlarged bladder in the second trimester is usually due to bladder outlet (urethral) obstruction. The presence of normal kidneys suggests that the renal function is likely to be preserved, and is usually confirmed with the additional finding of normal liquor volume. The latter is likely to be due to intermittent/partial outlet obstruction and tends to do well postnatally.

Obstructive uropathy

With posterior urethral valves, there is usually a more severe obstruction of the urethra, resulting in an enlarged and hypertrophied bladder with varying degrees of hydroureter and hydronephrosis, and a spectrum of renal hypoplasia/dysplasia, oligohydramnios, and pulmonary hypoplasia. In some cases, there is associated urinary ascites from rupture of the bladder or transudation of urine into the peritoneal cavity. The combination of an enlarged bladder with abnormal kidneys and reduced or absent liquor volume is indicative of poor renal function, and is generally indicative of poor prognosis.

Bibliography

1. Johnson MP, Freedman AL. Fetal uropathy. Curr Opin Obstet Gynecol 1999; 11(2): 185–94.
2. Liao AW, Sebire NJ, Geerts L, Cicero S, Nicolaides KH. Megacystis at 10–14 weeks of gestation: chromosomal defects and outcome according to bladder length. Ultrasound Obstet Gynecol 2003; 21(4): 338–41.
3. Robyr R, Benachi A, Daikha-Dahmane F et al. Correlation between ultrasound and anatomical findings in fetuses with lower urinary tract obstruction in the first half of pregnancy. Ultrasound Obstet Gynecol 2005; 25(5): 478–82.

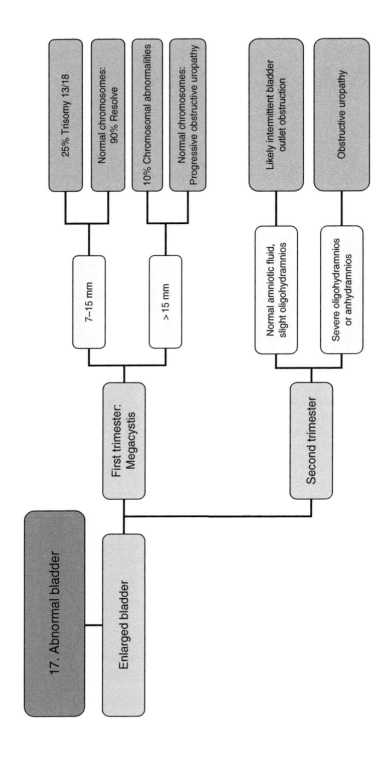

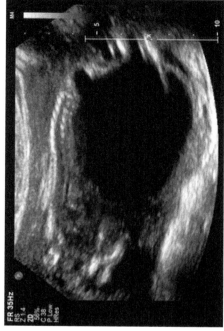

Fig. 17.1 *Megacystis*

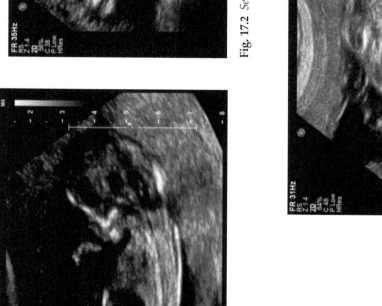

Fig. 17.2 *Severe obstructive uropathy*

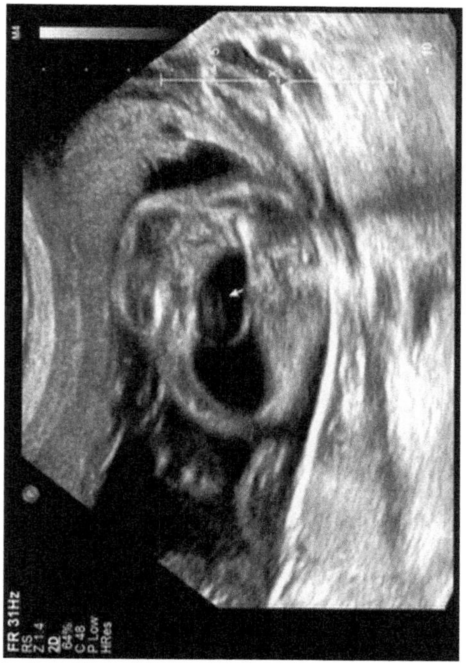

Fig. 17.3 *Cystocele*

18

SHORT FEMUR LENGTH

Shortened femur length is the commonest presentation for suspected skeletal problems, as this is the only bone that is routinely measured in obstetric ultrasound. In the majority of cases, shortening of the long bones is likely to represent inaccurate dating, constitutional smallness, or an early feature of fetal growth restriction. The latter must be excluded before contemplating a diagnosis of a fetal skeletal dysplasia, a heterogeneous group of disorders characterized by abnormalities of cartilage and bone growth. Typically, a diagnosis of a fetal skeletal dysplasia before 24 weeks results in a poor outcome due to thoracic dysplasia.

Fetal growth restriction

Approximately 10–15% of short femur lengths noted at the 20–22 week anomaly scan will subsequently turn out to be due to severe early onset fetal growth restriction secondary to placental insufficiency. The finding of notched, high-resistance uterine artery Doppler indices is characteristic of this diagnosis.

Fetal aneuploidy

Short femur length is a marker for chromosomal abnormality. A thorough search for associated markers of aneuploidy should be undertaken.

Normal bone modelling (< 24 weeks)

Unilateral femoral shortening is suggestive of focal femoral hypoplasia syndromes. Typically the prognosis is good in most of these syndromes. The finding of bilateral shortening is suggestive of achondrogenesis. The latter is a uniformly lethal condition associated with micromelia (extreme shortening of the entire limb) and thoracic dystrophy.

Abnormal bone modelling (< 24 weeks)

Bowing may be difficult to differentiate from fractures of the long bones, but both suggest the diagnoses of achondrogenesis, thanatophoric dysplasia, campomelic dysplasia, or osteogenesis imperfecta. Definitive hypomineralization is indicative of either hypophosphatasia or osteogenesis imperfecta. Polydactyly is characteristic of short-ribbed polydactyly at this gestation, and microcephaly occurs in chondrodysplasia punctata.

Third trimester diagnosis

The commonest diagnosis in the third trimester is achondroplasia (classical dwarfism). Spondyloepiphyseal dysplasia congenita (SEDC) is an alternative diagnosis, but this is rarely made prenatally as the ultrasound features are subtle. The presence of polydactyly is suggestive of Jeune dystrophy or Ellis–van Creveld syndrome.

Bibliography

1. Krakow D, Williams J 3rd, Poehl M, Rimoin DL, Platt LD. Use of three-dimensional ultrasound imaging in the diagnosis of prenatal-onset skeletal dysplasias. Ultrasound Obstet Gynecol 2003; 21(5): 467–72.
2. Lachman RS, Rappaport V. Fetal imaging in the skeletal dysplasias. Clin Perinatol 1990; 17(3): 703–22.

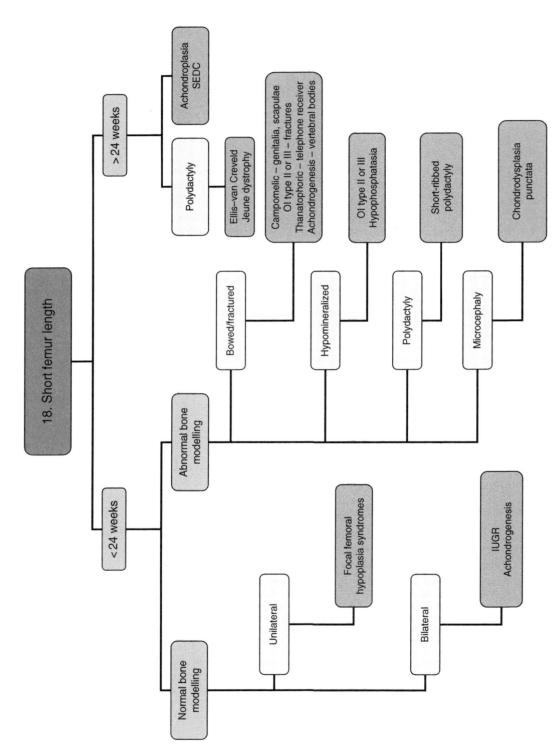

IUGR, intrauterine growth restriction; SEDC, spondyloepiphyseal dysplasia congenita; OI, osteogenesis imperfecta.

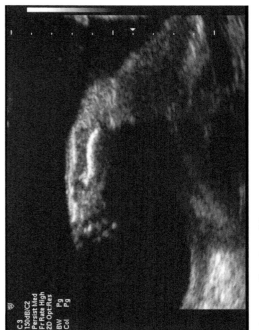

Fig. 18.1 *Short bowed femur*

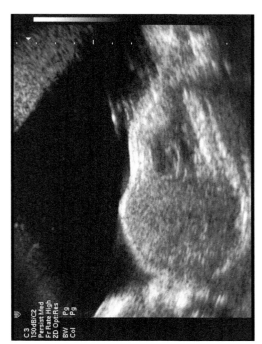

Fig. 18.2 *Short bowed forearm*

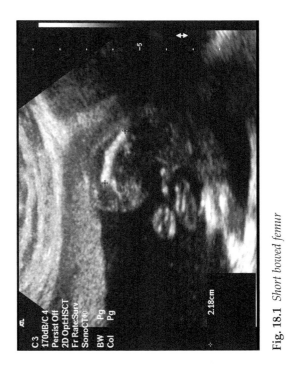

Fig. 18.3 *Short fractured femur*

Fig. 18.4 *Thoracic dystrophy*

19

JOINT ABNORMALITIES

Typically, joint abnormalities are only diagnosed prenatally when they are severe. However, false positive diagnosis may be made due to the natural joint mobility of fetuses, and the effect of uterine crowding due to advanced pregnancy, oligohydramnios, or multiple pregnancy.

Talipes

This is a varus deformity of the foot, which when diagnosed antenatally is due to abnormal innervation of the mucles of the ankle joint. When unilateral and isolated, the prognosis is very good. A significant proportion of complex/bilateral cases are associated with chromosomal abnormality, genetic syndromes, or neurodevelopmental disorders.

Fixed flexion of multiple joints

These findings fall under the umbrella term arthrogryposis multiplex congenita, which covers many different neuromuscular disorders with guarded postnatal prognoses. The finding of cutaneous webs at the joints is typical of multiple pterygium syndrome. The confinement of abnormalities to the lower limb with an abrupt spinal termination is characteristic of caudal regression syndrome, often associated with diabetic pregnancy. If abnormalities in long bone length, mineralization, or fractures are seen, a skeletal dysplasia should be suspected.

Abnormal tone/posture

Rarely, abnormal posture or tone may be noted in the fetal joints, suggesting a neuromuscular disorder, such as Pena–Shokeir sequence. The latter should only be suspected if the posture is persistently abnormal on several scans on different occasions.

Bibliography

1. Bakalis S, Sairam S, Homfray T et al. Outcome of antenatally diagnosed talipes equinovarus in an unselected obstetric population. Ultrasound Obstet Gynecol 2002; 20(3): 226–9.
2. Bonilla-Musoles F, Machado LE, Osborne NG. Multiple congenital contractures (congenital multiple arthrogryposis). J Perinat Med 2002; 30(1): 99–104.

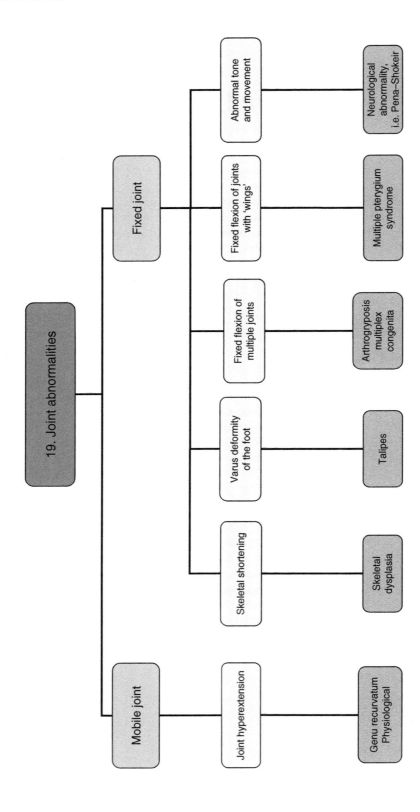

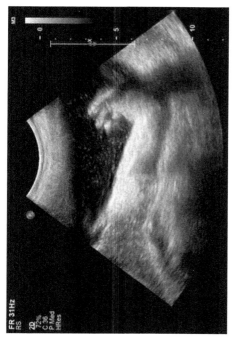

Fig. 19.2 *Wrist contracture*

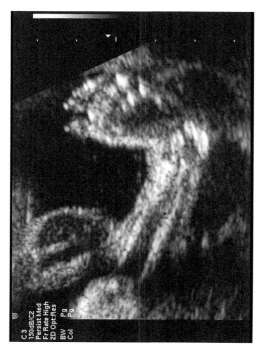

Fig. 19.1 *Talipes*

20

HAND ABNORMALITIES

Typically, abnormalities of the hand are only noted as part of a careful fetal survey after the diagnosis of another abnormality. Under these circumstances, the hand abnormalities are likely to be related to the chromosomal or genetic abnormality diagnosed.

Abnormal hand movement/posture

The presence of overlapping fingers or a clenched hand is suggestive of a chromosomal disorder such as trisomy 18 or a neuromuscular disorder such as Pena–Shokeir syndrome. If the hand is held in a decerebrate, inwardly turned posture, a radial array defect or neurodevelopmental problem should be suspected.

Abnormal hand structure

Polydactyly is a common isolated finding with an excellent prognosis. Associated features suggest a diagnosis such as a trisomy, skeletal dysplasia, Meckel–Gruber, and Smith–Lemli–Opitz syndrome. Missing or prematurely foreshortened digits are characteristic of amniotic band syndrome and terminal transverse limb defects. A split-hand or 'lobster-claw' deformity is suggestive of ectrodactyly.

Bibliography

1. Bromley B, Shipp TD, Benacerraf B. Isolated polydactyly: prenatal diagnosis and perinatal outcome. Prenat Diagn 2000; 20(11): 905–8.
2. Watson S. The principles of management of congenital anomalies of the upper limb. Arch Dis Child 2000; 83(1): 10–17.

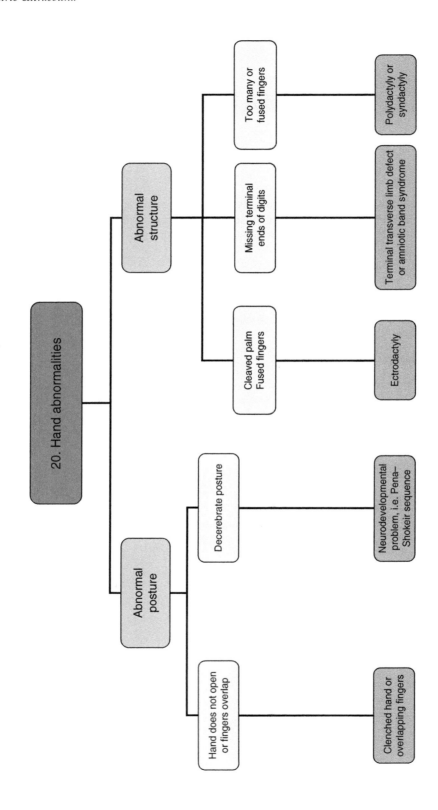

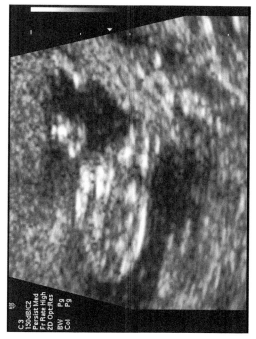

Fig. 20.2 *Ectrodactyly of the foot*

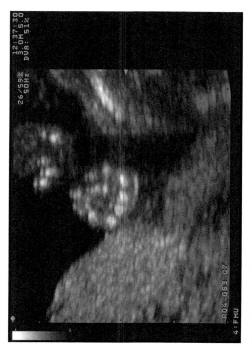

Fig. 20.1 *Overlapping fingers*

21

SPINAL ABNORMALITIES

The commonest spinal abnormality encountered prenatally is spina bifida. Although other spinal lesions are possible, they are relatively infrequent.

Spina bifida

Typically this is diagnosed on detection of the characteristic 'lemon-shaped' head and 'banana' cerebellum. The level of the lesion, the number of segments involved, and severity of the kyphoscoliosis, ventriculomegaly, and microcephaly determine the prognosis for the neonate.

Sacrococcygeal teratoma

This usually presents as a vascular, semi-solid/semi-cystic tumour at the terminal end of the spine. Sacrococcygeal teratomas are associated with fetal hydrops and polyhydramnios from high-output cardiac failure related to the arterio-venous shunting within the tumour. These tumours are only rarely malignant, and the prognosis tends to be good after resection.

Spinal angulation

Hemivertebrae are rarely diagnosed prenatally, probably because of the low prevalence and the relatively difficult ultrasound diagnosis. Most cases have a good prognosis, but consideration should be given to the diagnosis of VATER (vertebral, anal, tracheo-(o)esophageal, (o)esophageal, renal) or VACTERL (as above, plus cardiac, limb) associations. Kyphosis (exaggerated hump) and scoliosis (lateral deformity) may be diagnosed prenatally as isolated abnormalities. Occasionally they may be associated with spina bifida, body stalk abnormality, and skeletal dysplasias.

Caudal regression

This can vary in severity from partial sacral agenesis to complete absence of the lumbosacral spine. In an extreme form (sirenomelia), it presents with fusion and hypoplasia of the lower extremities and pelvic structures. Caudal regression occurs more commonly in diabetic pregnancy.

Bibliography

1. Mitchell LE, Adzick NS, Melchionne J et al. Spina bifida. Lancet 2004; 364(9448): 1885–95.
2. Nyberg DA. The fetal central nervous system. Semin Roentgenol 1990; 25(4): 317–33.

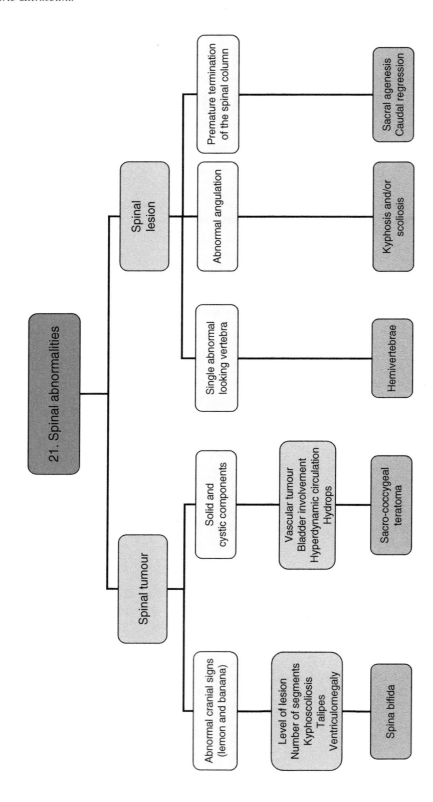

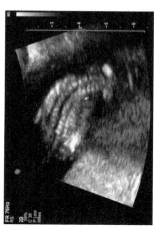

Fig. 21.5 *Kyphoscoliosis*

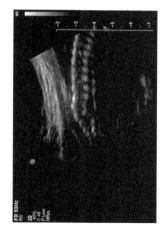
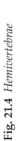

Fig. 21.6 *Caudal regression*

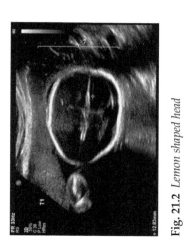

Fig. 21.2 *Lemon shaped head*

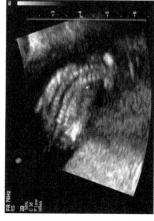
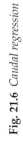

Fig. 21.3 *Banana cerebellum*

Fig. 21.4 *Hemivertebrae*

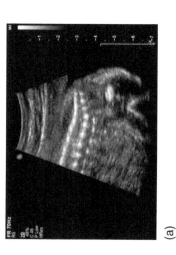

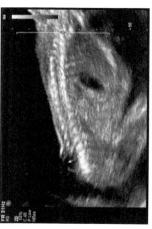
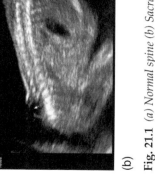

Fig. 21.1 *(a) Normal spine (b) Sacral meningomyelocele*

22

HEAD AND NECK MASSES

Fetal head and neck tumours are rare. The prognosis of these tumours largely depends on their size. If they are large they can cause compression of the trachea and neonatal airway, requiring ex-utero intrapartum treatment (EXIT) delivery. Fetal hydrops in highly vascular tumours and polyhydramnios due to poor swallowing are both associated with poorer outcomes.

Cervical teratoma

This is a very rare embryonic tumour of the neck with a heterogeneous appearance on ultrasound. They are usually unilateral, solid/cystic, multiloculated masses measuring 5–12 cm, commonly seen with calcifications.

Epignathus

This is a very rare mature teratoma of the oro-pharyngeal region, which presents as a solid tumour of the oral and/or nasal cavities usually associated with polyhydramnios. The tumour is often very vascular, and this can lead to fetal cardiac decompensation and hydrops. The anatomy of the brain must be carefully examined as intracranial extension can occur.

Fetal goitre

This is enlargement of the fetal thyroid gland. It can be due to maternal thyroid disease, but has also been reported in euthyroid women. Ultrasound features are of a symmetrical anterior solid mass which can result in hyperextension of the fetal head.

Cystic hygroma

This is the commonest cause for a fetal neck mass, and is thought to be due to lymphatic malformation. In the first trimester, cystic hygromas can be identified as increased nuchal translucency at the 11–13 + 6 week scan. Second trimester diagnosis is by an ultrasound finding of a thin-walled cystic swelling at the back of the neck with a characteristic midline septum (the nuchal ligament), often with multiple septa. Fetal cystic hygromas are strongly associated with underlying chromosomal abnormalities and genetic syndromes.

Fetal haemangioma

Fetal haemangioma affecting the neck or face is a rare condition, and appears as a thick-walled sonolucent mass with characteristic pulsating Doppler flow signals.

Ex-utero intrapartum treatment (EXIT)

The aim of the procedure is to allow time to secure the airway in the newborn while maintaining uteroplacental gas exchange at Caesarean section. This is achieved by endotracheal intubation or tracheostomy while still connected to the placenta.

Bibliography

1. Chervenak FA, Isaacson G, Touloukian R et al. Diagnosis and management of fetal teratomas. Obstet Gynecol 1985; 66: 666–71.
2. Gallagher PG, Mahoney MJ, Gosche JR. Cystic hygroma in the fetus and newborn. Semin Perinatol 1999; 23(4): 341–56.
3. Nicolaides KH. Nuchal translucency and other first-trimester sonographic markers of aneuploidy. Am J Obstet Gynecol 2004; 191: 45–67.

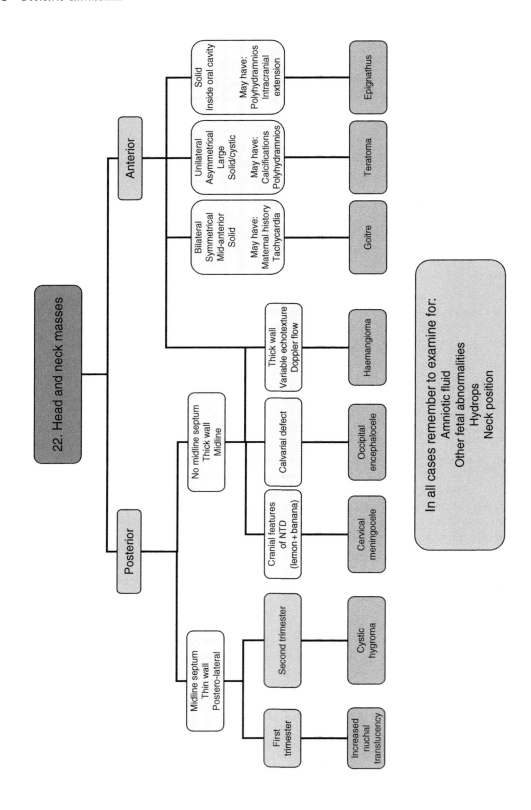

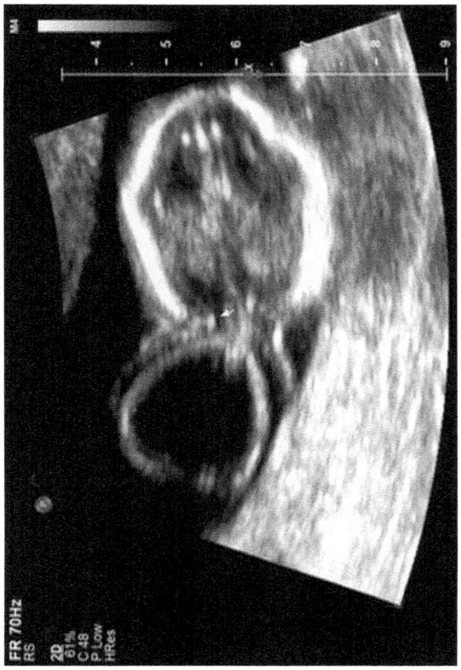

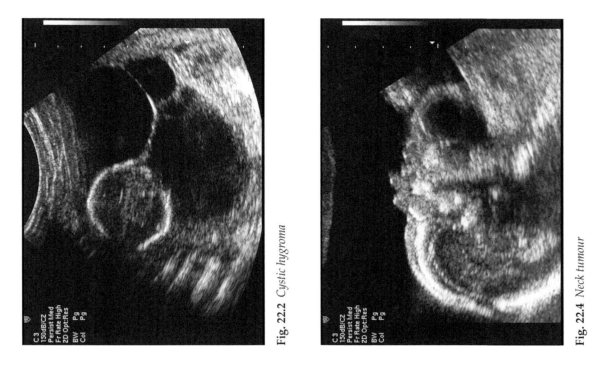

Fig. 22.1 *Encephalocele*

Fig. 22.2 *Cystic hygroma*

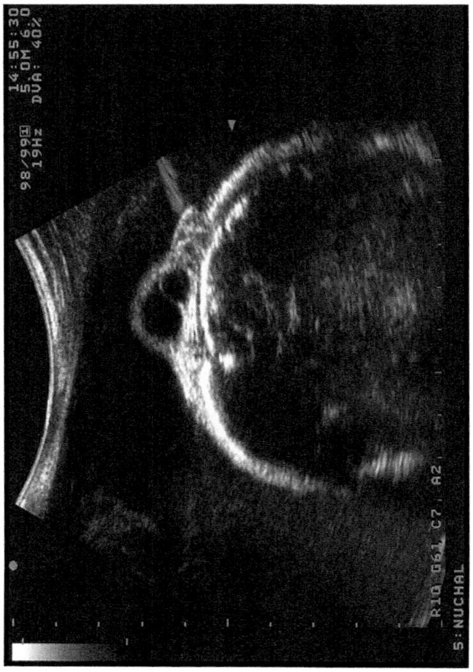

Fig. 22.3 *Facial cyst*

Fig. 22.4 *Neck tumour*

23

INCREASED NUCHAL TRANSLUCENCY

All fetuses have a collection of fluid under the skin behind the neck at 11–13 + 6 weeks of gestation. This nuchal translucency (NT) is visible and measurable on ultrasound. There are many causes of increased NT, and there may not be a single underlying mechanism for its presence.

Chromosomal abnormalities

Nuchal translucency (NT) is the single most important marker for chromosomal abnormalities in the first trimester, and by far the most widely researched. Screening for trisomy 21 by combining NT with maternal age results in a detection rate of about 80% for a 5% invasive testing rate. The NT is increased in other chromosomal abnormalities, and a screening programme for trisomy 21 will also detect the majority of fetuses with other trisomies. Combining NT screening with other first-trimester ultrasound markers (nasal bone, ductus venosus, tricuspid regurgitation) as well as first- and second-trimester maternal serum markers increases the detection rate of chromosomal defects further.

Cardiac defects

Heart abnormalities are associated with increased NT thickness in chromosomally normal fetuses. The prevalence of heart abnormalities is about 7% if the NT is 4.5–5.4 mm, 20% for NT of 5.5–6.4 mm, and 30% for NT of 6.5 mm or more. Using NT as a screening test for major heart defects will significantly improve detection rates for cardiac abnormalities. In pregnancies with increased NT, specialist fetal echocardiography should be considered for fetuses with an NT above the 95th centile.

Fetal abnormalities and movement disorders

Increased fetal NT is associated with a high prevalence of major fetal abnormalities. There is a long and growing list of abnormalities associated with increased NT, and common defects include hydrops, congenital diaphragmatic hernia, exomphalos, body stalk anomaly, skeletal abnormalities, and fetal movement disorders such as fetal akinesia deformation sequence. A careful anatomical survey should therefore be performed in chromosomally normal fetuses with increased NT, and this should include looking for normal fetal movements.

Genetic syndromes

Increased NT has been associated with a large number of genetic syndromes. The rarity of these means that it can be difficult to establish whether the observed prevalence is higher than in the general population, but it appears that congenital adrenal hyperplasia, fetal akinesia deformation sequence, Noonan syndrome, Smith–Lemli–Opitz syndrome, and spinal muscular atrophy are more prevalent than expected in the general population.

Bibliography

1. Makrydimas G, Sotiriadis A, Huggon IC et al. Nuchal translucency and fetal cardiac defects: a pooled analysis of major fetal echocardiography centers. Am J Obstet Gynecol 2005; 192(1): 89–95.
2. Snijders RJ, Noble P, Sebire N, Souka A, Nicolaides KH. UK multicentre project on assessment of risk of trisomy 21 by maternal age and fetal nuchal-translucency thickness at 10–14 weeks of gestation. Fetal Medicine Foundation First Trimester Screening Group. Lancet 1998; 352(9125): 343–6.
3. www.fetalmedicine.com.

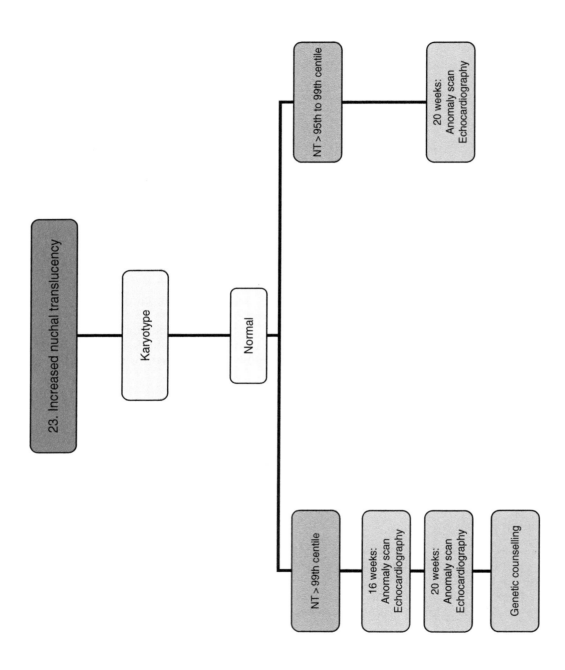

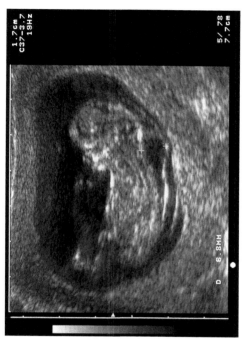

Fig. 23.2 *Increased nuchal measurement*

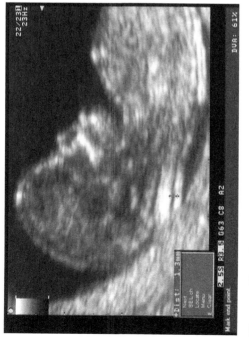

Fig. 23.1 *Normal nuchal measurement*

24

PLACENTAL ABNORMALITIES

Molar pregnancy

Hydatidiform mole can be divided into complete (where there is no fetus) and partial/incomplete (where a fetus is present). Ultrasound shows the placenta to be an enlarged complex intrauterine mass containing many small cysts which can be described as grape-like (hydatidiform). The classic image of a snowstorm pattern can sometimes be seen, but the description is based on older ultrasound technology.

Chorioangiomas

These are benign vascular tumours which rarely can result in fetal complications such as cardiomegaly, polyhydramnios, anaemia, hydrops, and occasionally fetal growth restriction. Targeted ultrasound using colour Doppler can help in identifying chorioangiomas in cases with the latter complications.

Placental cysts

These are seen just beneath the chorionic plate and are of no apparent clinical significance. They are thought to be caused by the deposition of fibrin in the intervillous space.

Placental lakes

Placental lakes appear as sonolucent areas in the placenta. They are often seen in cases of fetal growth restriction due to placental insufficiency. However, they are poor in the prediction of uteroplacental insufficiency as they are commonly seen in normal pregnancy, especially with advancing gestation.

Jelly-like placenta

Rarely the placenta can appear thick, with patches of decreased echogenicity. Jelly-like refers to the placenta quivering like jelly in response to sharp abdominal pressure. The finding has been reported as being strongly associated with an adverse pregnancy outcome. In such cases it may therefore be advisable to perform serial growth scans.

Placental grading

Placental grading was used in order to identify pregnancies at risk of fetal growth restriction before the wide availability of Doppler equipment. In addition, the poor correlation of placental grade to neonatal outcome has meant that the effectiveness of reporting Grannum grades in clinical practice is limited and largely historical.

Placenta accreta

In this condition the placenta is adherent to the uterus, and should be suspected in cases of placenta praevia or previous Caesarean section. Ultrasound features include a loss of the hypoechoic area between placenta and myometrium, large intraplacental lakes, or irregular vascular sinuses with turbulent flow within the placenta.

Bibliography

1. Harris RD, Cho C, Wells WA. Sonography of the placenta with emphasis on pathological correlation. Semin Ultrasound CT MR 1996; 17(1): 66–89.
2. Thompson MO, Vines SK, Aquilina J, Wathen NC, Harrington K. Are placental lakes of any clinical significance? Placenta 2002; 23(8–9): 685–90.

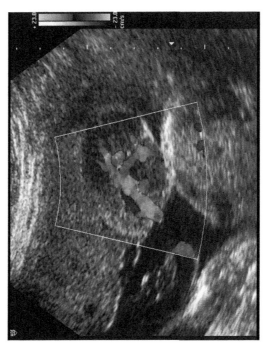

Fig. 24.2 *Placental chorioangioma (see also colour plate)*

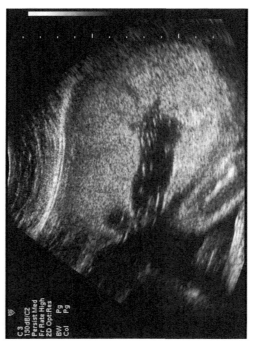

Fig. 24.1 *Placenta lakes*

25

SINGLE UMBILICAL ARTERY

The normal umbilical cord contains two arteries and one vein. A single umbilical artery occurs in around 1% of cords in singletons, but the incidence may be higher in women with diabetes, and lower in those of African and Japanese ethnic origin. The antenatal diagnosis can be by examination of a transverse section of the cord using B mode, or by using colour Doppler to image the origin of the umbilical arteries on each side of the fetal bladder.

Chromosomal abnormalities

About 20–30% of fetuses with a single umbilical artery have associated abnormalities, usually chromosomal (trisomy and triploidy). The commonly reported defects are cardiac, abdominal wall, and urinary tract abnormalities.

Isolated two-vessel cord

In a low-risk patient, the finding of an isolated single umbilical artery does not significantly increase the risk for a chromosomal defect. In isolated cases, the perinatal morbidity may be increased due to the association of fetal growth restriction in 10–15% of cases.

Management

Prenatal diagnosis of a single umbilical artery should prompt careful examination for other abnormalities, and fetal karyotyping should be considered if these are found. In ongoing cases serial ultrasound examination to ensure linear fetal growth should be performed.

Bibliography

1. Cristina MP, Ana G, Ines T, Manuel GE, Enrique IG. Perinatal results following the prenatal ultrasound diagnosis of single umbilical artery. Acta Obstet Gynecol Scand 2005; 84(11): 1068–74.
2. Predanic M, Perni SC, Friedman A, Chervenak FA, Chasen ST. Fetal growth assessment and neonatal birth weight in fetuses with an isolated single umbilical artery. Obstet Gynecol 2005; 105(5 Pt 1): 1093–7.

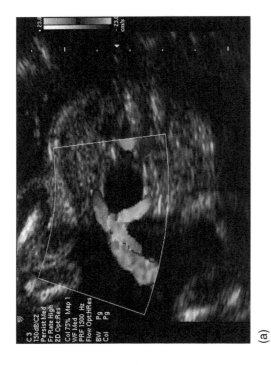

(a)

(b)

Fig. 25.2 *(a) Two umbilical arteries on colour Doppler (b) Single umbilical artery on colour Doppler (see also colour plate)*

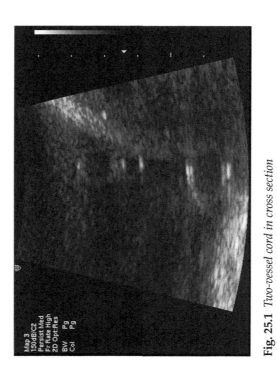

Fig. 25.1 *Two-vessel cord in cross section*

26

OLIGOHYDRAMNIOS

Oligohydramnios occurs in 0.5–1% of pregnancies. The diagnosis is usually made subjectively. It is defined as an amniotic fluid index (AFI) of less than 5 cm or a deepest single pocket measurement of 1 cm or less. Oligo-anhydramnios is caused because there is reduced production of fetal urine (e.g. placental insufficiency, renal agenesis), or because the fetus cannot urinate due to an obstruction (e.g. posterior urethral valves), or because the fluid that is produced drains away due to rupture of the membranes (ROM). Anhydramnios means that no amniotic fluid is seen. With anhydramnios there is marked fetal deformation due to fetal compression, including a flattened face, hypertelorism, low-set ears, and micrognathia (Potter syndrome).

Preterm prelabour rupture of membranes

Amniotic fluid is mainly produced by fetal urine, but before 16 weeks the placenta contributes significantly. Therefore oligohydramnios is unusual before 16 weeks, with the exception of preterm prelabour rupture of the membranes (PPROM). Typically, however, this is a diagnosis of exclusion after all other causes have been deemed unlikely.

Renal tract abnormality

The absence of fluid and the associated abnormal posturing of the fetus can make examination for fetal abnormalities difficult. However, a dilated bladder in urethral obstruction and bilateral cystic kidneys are easily seen on ultrasound.

Fetal growth restriction

Fetal growth restriction can present with oligohydramnios. This should typically have the characteristic fetal and uterine Doppler profiles indicative of uteroplacental insufficiency.

Prognosis

The prognosis is usually poor with presentations before 24 weeks, mainly because a lack of amniotic fluid causes pulmonary hypoplasia due to compression of the chest and abdomen and limitation of movement of the diaphragm. Fetal compromise may also occur because of severe renal disease or severe fetal growth restriction. When thought to be idiopathic, the prognosis is generally good, with only a moderate increase in fetal and neonatal morbidity.

Bibliography

1. Newbould MJ, Lendon M, Barson AJ. Oligohydramnios sequence: the spectrum of renal malformations. Br J Obstet Gynaecol 1994; 101(7): 598–604.
2. Shipp TD, Bromley B, Pauker S, Frigoletto FD Jr, Benacerraf BR. Outcome of singleton pregnancies with severe oligohydramnios in the second and third trimesters. Ultrasound Obstet Gynecol 1996; 7(2): 108–13.

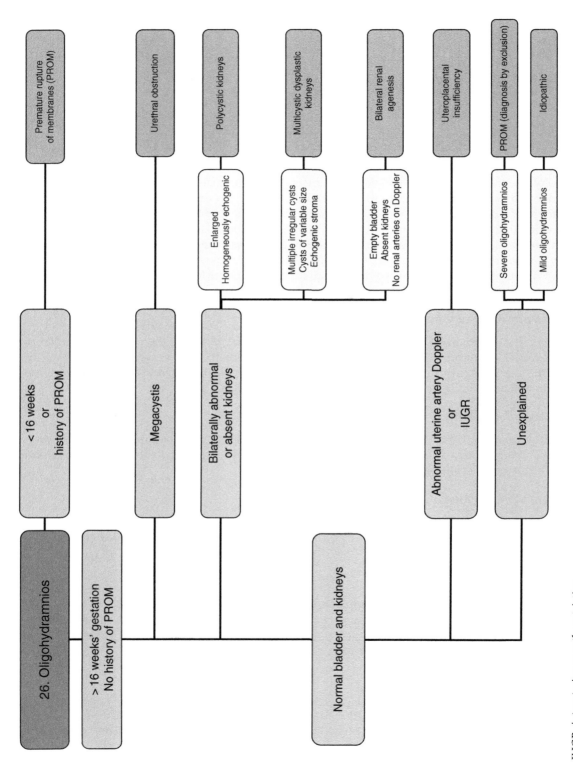

IUGR, intrauterine growth restriction.

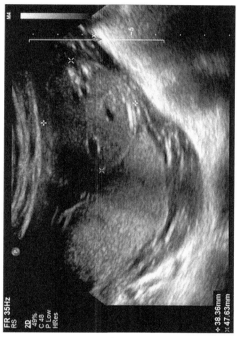

Fig. 26.1 *Anhydramnios*

27

POLYHYDRAMNIOS

Polyhydramnios is caused by reduced fetal swallowing, or increased fetal urine production. This occurs in 0.5–1% of pregnancies. The diagnosis is usually made subjectively, but it is defined as an amniotic fluid index (AFI) of more than 24 cm or a deepest single pocket measurement of fluid of at least 8 cm. If the deepest pool is greater than 11 cm it is termed moderate, and if more than 15 cm, severe polyhydramnios.

Prognosis

Even in the absence of fetal defects the perinatal mortality rate is about two to three times that of pregnancies with normal amniotic fluid volume. With a fetal or placental malformation the perinatal mortality is as high as 60%.

Twin–twin transfusion syndrome

By far the commonest cause of polyhydramnios in monochorionic twin pregnancy is twin–twin transfusion syndrome (TTTS). This is also one of the very few causes of polyhydramnios at less than 20 weeks of gestation.

Fetal structural abnormalities

Most defects are usually gastrointestinal or in the central nervous system. The presence of multiple abnormalities, or abnormalities that do not explain the polyhydramnios, should raise the suspicion of an underlying chromosomal or genetic syndrome.

Fetal movement disorders

Absent or greatly reduced fetal movement can be suggestive of neuromuscular disease, usually with a guarded postnatal prognosis.

Placental tumours

The presence of a placental tumour, such as a chorioangioma, may cause a hyperdynamic circulation, and subsequent hydrops.

Fetal anaemia

Typically, Doppler examination of the middle cerebral artery should reval a high peak systolic velocity. Fetal oedema, ascites, or hydrops may be present if the anaemia is severe.

Arrhythmias

Fetal supraventricular tachycardia or heart block can cause polyhydramnios and, subsequently, hydrops.

Bibliography

1. Biggio JR Jr, Wenstrom KD, Dubard MB, Cliver SP. Hydramnios prediction of adverse perinatal outcome. Obstet Gynecol 1999; 94(5 Pt 1): 773–7.
2. Desmedt EJ, Henry OA, Beischer NA. Polyhydramnios and associated maternal and fetal complications in singleton pregnancies. Br J Obstet Gynaecol 1990; 97(12): 1115–22.

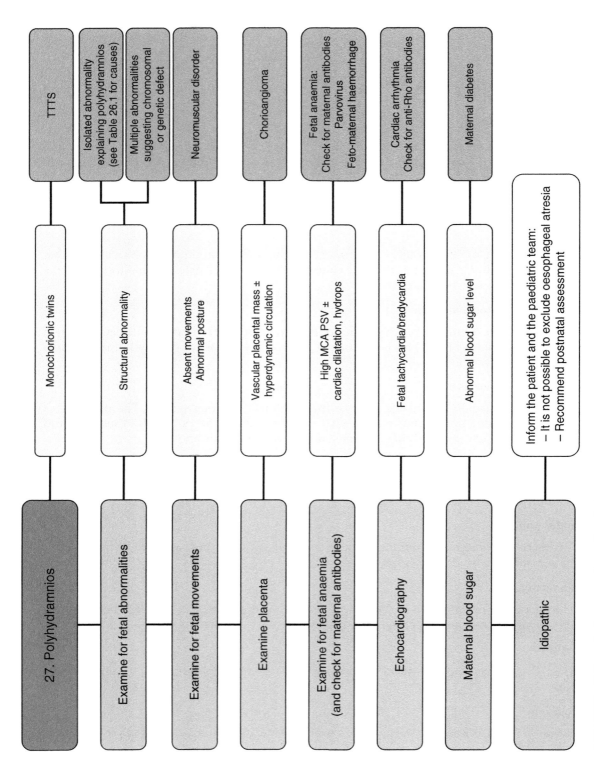

27. Polyhydramnios

Examine for fetal abnormalities
- Structural abnormality → Isolated abnormality explaining polyhydramnios (see Table 26.1 for causes) / Multiple abnormalities suggesting chromosomal or genetic defect
- Monochorionic twins → TTTS

Examine for fetal movements
- Absent movements / Abnormal posture → Neuromuscular disorder

Examine placenta
- Vascular placental mass ± hyperdynamic circulation → Chorioangioma

Examine for fetal anaemia (and check for maternal antibodies)
- High MCA PSV ± cardiac dilatation, hydrops → Fetal anaemia: Check for maternal antibodies / Parvovirus / Feto-maternal haemorrhage

Echocardiography
- Fetal tachycardia/bradycardia → Cardiac arrhythmia / Check for anti-Rho antibodies

Maternal blood sugar
- Abnormal blood sugar level → Maternal diabetes

Idiopathic
- Inform the patient and the paediatric team:
  – It is not possible to exclude oesophageal atresia
  – Recommend postnatal assessment

MCA PSV, middle cerebral artery peak systolic velocity; TTTS, twin–twin transfusion syndrome.

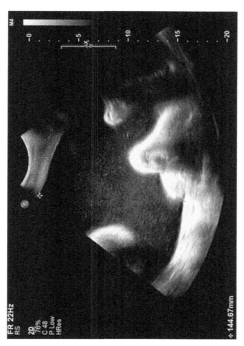

Fig. 27.1 *Polyhydramnios*

28

AMNIOTIC SHELF/BAND

Amniotic bands occur as a consequence of a disruption to the amnion, with an intact chorion. In most cases, amniotic bands occur without any associated fetal effects, although occasionally a diagnosis of amniotic band syndrome may be made. Amniotic band syndrome is believed to be caused by the entrapment of fetal parts (usually a limb or digits) in fibrous amniotic bands while in utero. When the amnion ruptures without injury to the chorion, the fetus comes in contact with free-floating sticky amniotic 'bands'. The amniotic bands can entangle various fetal parts, thereby reducing the blood supply and causing congenital abnormalities, typically amputations. Although no two cases are exactly alike, there are several features that are relatively common: syndactyly, distal ring constrictions, shortened bone growth, limb length discrepancy, distal lymphoedema, and congenital bands. Very confusingly, by the time amniotic band syndrome is suspected, the amniotic bands are no longer visible, as the fetal insult probably occurred early in the first trimester.

Bibliography

1. Lockwood C, Ghidini A, Romero R, Hobbins JC. Amniotic band syndrome: reevaluation of its pathogenesis. Am J Obstet Gynecol 1989; 160(5 Pt 1): 1030–3.
2. Seeds JW, Cefalo RC, Herbert WNP. Amniotic band syndrome. Am J Obstet Gynecol 1982; 144(3): 243–8.

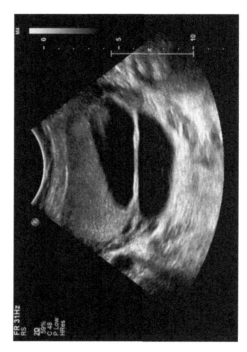

Fig. 28.1 *Amniotic band*

29

HYDROPS

Hydrops is defined as an abnormal accumulation of serous fluid in at least two fetal compartments, including ascites, pleural or pericardial effusions, and skin oedema. It is a rare finding and can be the result of cardiac failure, obstructed lymphatic flow, or decreased plasma osmotic pressure.

Monochorionic twin pregnancy

The finding of hydrops in one monochorionic twin is typical of either twin–twin transfusion or twin reversed arterial perfusion syndrome.

Hyperdynamic circulation

The finding of a high peak systolic velocity on middle cerebral artery Doppler is suggestive of hyperdynamic heart failure as the cause of hydrops. The presence of a fetal or placental tumour can cause this by creating an arterio-venous shunt within the fetal circulation. In the absence of a tumour, fetal anaemia is the most likely cause secondary to red blood cell allo-immunization, parvovirus infection, or feto-maternal haemorrhage, or due to inherited fetal anaemias.

Fetal structural abnormality

Cardiac failure as a consequence of congenital heart defects and arrhythmias is the commonest cause of hydrops in this group. The other reason for hydrops is thoracic compression leading to cardiac failure. Typically, the fetal abnormalities associated with this are cystic adenomatoid malformation and diaphragmatic hernia.

Fetal syndromes

These include chromosomal (trisomy and Turner syndrome), genetic (Noonan syndrome), and metabolic disorders (glycogen storage diseases, lysosome storage diseases).

Fetal congenital infections

These are most commonly due to early pregnancy congenital infection with cytomegalovirus, toxoplasmosis, coxsackievirus, or *Listeria*.

Bibliography

1. Bukowski R, Saade GR. Hydrops fetalis. Clin Perinatol 2000; 27(4): 1007–31.
2. Sohan K, Carroll SG, De La Fuente S, Soothill P, Kyle P. Analysis of outcome in hydrops fetalis in relation to gestational age at diagnosis, cause and treatment. Acta Obstet Gynecol Scand 2001; 80(8): 726–30.

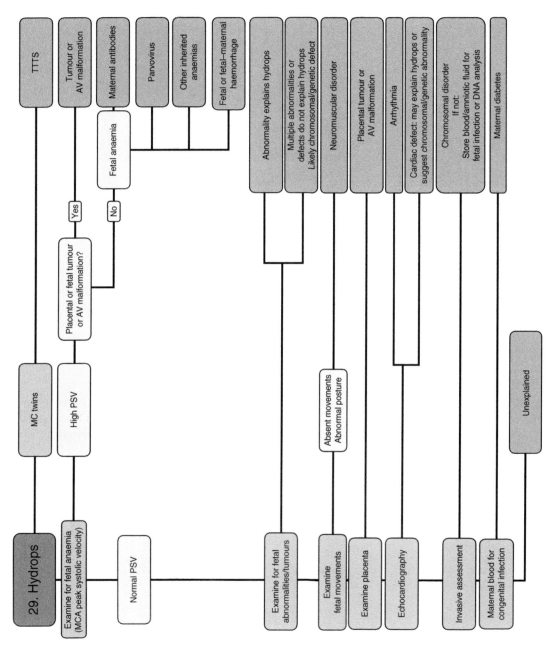

MCA, middle cerebral artery; PSV, peak systolic velocity; MC, monochorionic; AV, arterio-venous; TTTS, twin–twin transfusion syndrome.

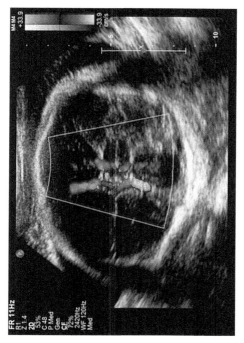

Fig. 29.2 *Middle cerebral artery colour Doppler (see also colour plate)*

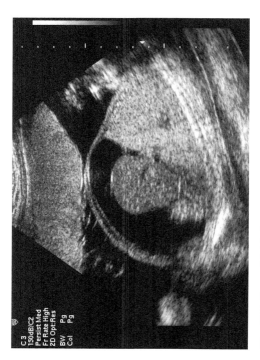

Fig. 29.1 *Severe fetal hydrops*

30

SMALL FETUS

Fetal growth restriction (FGR) is defined as growth below the 5th centile for gestational age. Broadly speaking, there are four causes for this finding: incorrect dating, constitutionally small fetus, placental insufficiency, or fetal abnormality.

Incorrect dating

1. Check the pregnancy history for a previous dating scan. Earlier scans will be more reliable, particularly if done between 10 and 14 weeks. **Once the pregnancy has been dated in this way, do not change the gestational age again.**
2. If no previous scans are available, date by the last menstrual period (LMP).
3. In cases where pregnancies are dated late or there is a question regarding the gestation, a scan in 3–4 weeks should be performed to ensure that fetal growth continues on the same centile. If there is a further fall in growth, consider an alternative diagnosis.

Constitutionally small baby

1. The mother and/or father may be of small stature.
2. Previous babies have been small for gestational age.
3. Be aware of ethnic differences in birth weight.
4. A follow-up growth scan will often show a slight fall from the centile line.
5. The uterine and fetal Doppler studies are entirely normal.

Placental insufficiency

1. Previous pregnancies may have been affected by placental insufficiency, pre-eclampsia, or placental abruption.
2. FGR is asymmetrical. In general, the abdominal circumference is smaller than the head circumference. In some cases of severe early onset growth restriction, femur length may be the first index to be affected. Doppler studies are abnormal, with the usual sequence of abnormal Doppler waveforms present first in the uterine, then the umbilical, and then the middle cerebral arteries.

Fetal abnormality

1. The presence of FGR in the presence of fetal structural abnormalities, markers for chromosomal defects, or polyhydramnios makes the presence of congenital or aquired fetal abnormality likely.
2. Causes include: chromosomal abnormality, congenital fetal infection, fetal alcohol syndrome, and genetic abnormality (e.g. uniparental disomy, Silver–Russell syndrome).

Bibliography

1. Baschat AA. Pathophysiology of fetal growth restriction: implications for diagnosis and surveillance. Obstet Gynecol Surv 2004; 59(8): 617–27.
2. Baschat AA, Galan HL, Bhide A et al. Doppler and biophysical assessment in growth restricted fetuses: distribution of test results. Ultrasound Obstet Gynecol 2006; 27(1): 41–7.

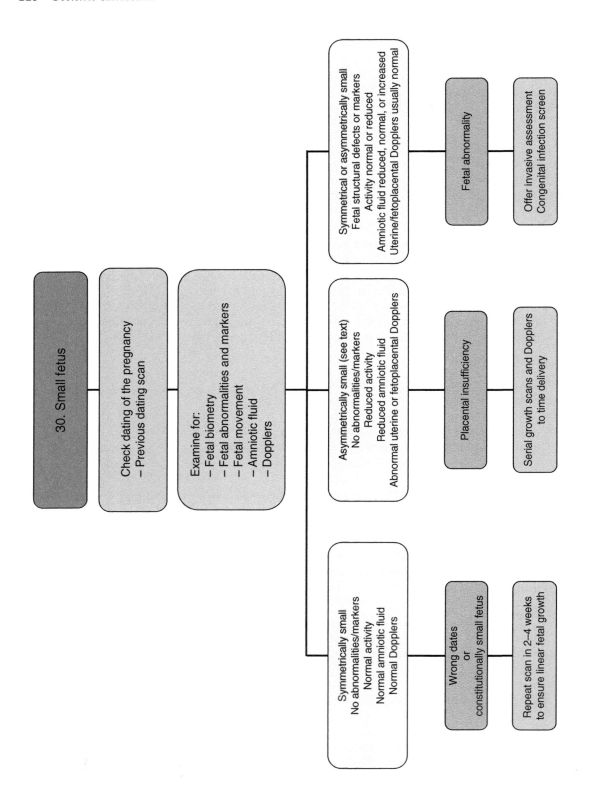

30. Small fetus

Check dating of the pregnancy
– Previous dating scan

Examine for:
– Fetal biometry
– Fetal abnormalities and markers
– Fetal movement
– Amniotic fluid
– Dopplers

Symmetrically small
No abnormalities/markers
Normal activity
Normal amniotic fluid
Normal Dopplers

Wrong dates
or
constitutionally small fetus

Repeat scan in 2–4 weeks
to ensure linear fetal growth

Asymmetrically small (see text)
No abnormalities/markers
Reduced activity
Reduced amniotic fluid
Abnormal uterine or fetoplacental Dopplers

Placental insufficiency

Serial growth scans and Dopplers
to time delivery

Symmetrical or asymmetrically small
Fetal structural defects or markers
Activity normal or reduced
Amniotic fluid reduced, normal, or increased
Uterine/fetoplacental Dopplers usually normal

Fetal abnormality

Offer invasive assessment
Congenital infection screen

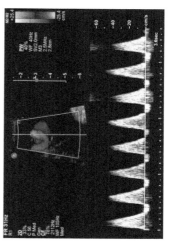

Fig. 30.2 *Absent end-diastolic flow in the umbilical artery (see also colour plate)*

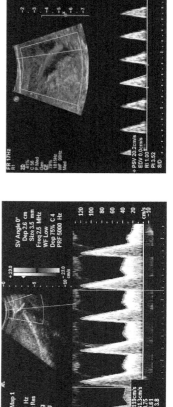

Fig. 30.1 *High resistance uterine artery Doppler (see also colour plate)*

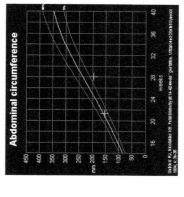

Fig. 30.3 *Reversed end-diastolic flow in the umbilical artery (see also colour plate)*

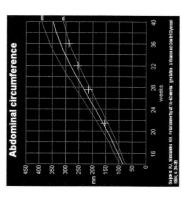

Fig. 30.6 *Growth velocity in placental insufficiency*

Fig. 30.5 *Normally small growth velocity*

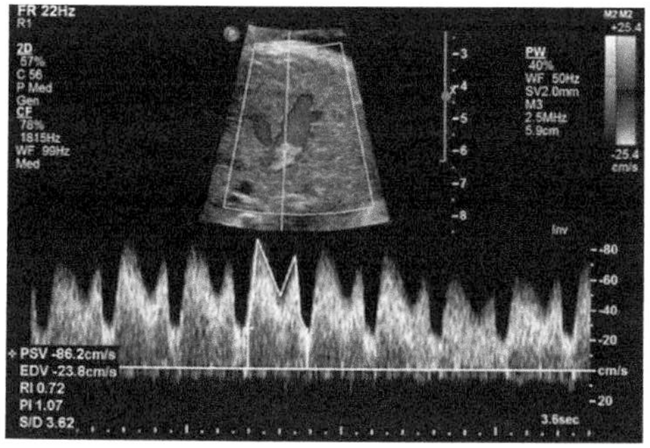

Fig. 30.4 *High resistance ductus venosus Doppler (see also colour plate)*

31

TWIN–TWIN TRANSFUSION SYNDROME

About 10–15% of monochorionic (MC) twin pregnancies are complicated by severe twin–twin transfusion syndrome (TTTS) as a consequence of a chronic circulatory imbalance in the vascular anastomoses that occur in virtually all MC placentae. TTTS typically presents in the mid-second trimester. The diagnosis is based on the donor presenting with oligo-anhydramnios and the recipient having polyhydramnios. The donor appears to be stuck, with restricted growth and an absent/small bladder. The recipient appears to be of average/increased weight with a big bladder. Doppler changes may accompany these findings and usually signify worsening TTTS. The donor twin may have absent/reversed end-diastolic flow in the umbilical artery. The recipient and, less commonly, the donor may show absent or reversed flow during atrial contraction in the ductus venosus.

Staging of twin–twin transfusion syndrome

The natural history of TTTS has been classified into five stages (Table 31.1). The differential diagnoses from TTTS are much rarer, and include acute inter-twin transfusion and selective fetal growth restriction.

Acute inter-twin transfusion

Acute inter-twin transfusion usually occurs as a consequence of an acute vascular imbalance in previously healthy MC twins. It presents in the late second or third trimester with acute polyhydramnios in normally grown MC twins. Amniodrainage may be required to reduce the risk of preterm labour from the polyhydramnios, and in the majority of cases the symptoms do not recur.

Selective fetal growth restriction

This presents in the second trimester with one growth restricted twin (as in TTTS) and one apparently healthy, normally grown twin. The majority of cases can be managed conservatively, but fetoscopic laser may sometimes be required if preterm death of the growth restricted twin seems likely.

Table 31.1 *Natural history of twin–twin transfusion syndrome*

Stage	Poly-oligo hydramnios	Bladder in donor	Abnormal Dopplers	Hydrops	Demise
I	Yes	Yes	No	No	No
II	Yes	No	No	No	No
III	Yes	No	Yes	No	No
IV	Yes	No	Yes	Yes	No
V	Yes	No	Yes	Yes	Yes

Bibliography

1. Robyr R, Quarello E, Ville Y. Management of fetofetal transfusion syndrome. Prenat Diagn 2005; 25(9): 786–95.
2. Senat MV, Deprest J, Boulvain M et al. Endoscopic laser surgery versus serial amnioreduction for severe twin-to-twin transfusion syndrome. N Engl J Med 2004; 351: 136–44.

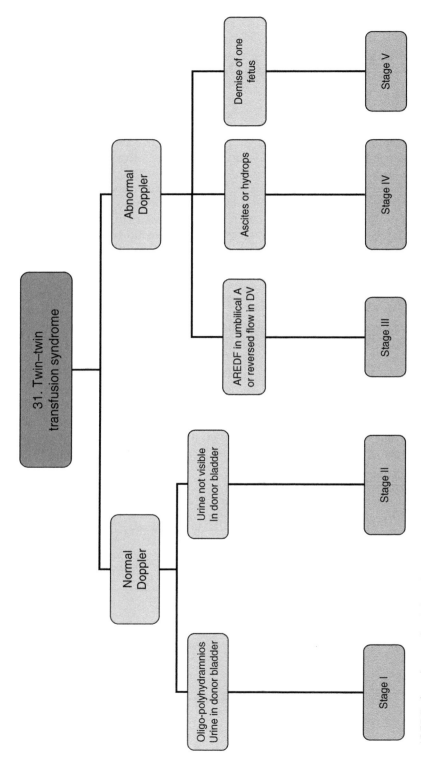

AREDF, absent/reversed end-diastolic flow; A, artery; DV, ductus venosus.

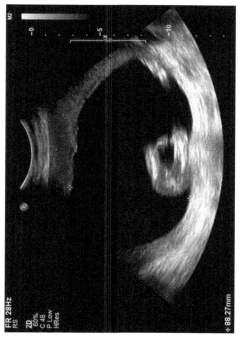

Fig. 31.1 *TTTS recipient with enlarged bladder*

INDEX

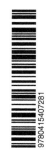